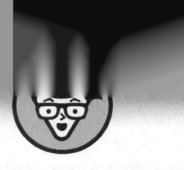

Macro Diet

by Malia Frey, MA, ACE-CPT, CHC

for
dummies®

A Wiley Brand

Macro Diet For Dummies®

Published by: **John Wiley & Sons, Inc.**, 111 River Street, Hoboken, NJ 07030-5774, www.wiley.com

Copyright © 2024 by John Wiley & Sons, Inc., Hoboken, New Jersey

Media and software compilation copyright © 2024 by John Wiley & Sons, Inc. All rights reserved.

Published simultaneously in Canada

For general information on our other products and services, please contact our Customer Care Department within the U.S. at 877-762-2974, outside the U.S. at 317-572-3993, or fax 317-572-4002. For technical support, please visit https://hub.wiley.com/community/support/dummies.

Wiley publishes in a variety of print and electronic formats and by print-on-demand. Some material included with standard print versions of this book may not be included in e-books or in print-on-demand. If this book refers to media such as a CD or DVD that is not included in the version you purchased, you may download this material at http://booksupport.wiley.com. For more information about Wiley products, visit www.wiley.com.

Library of Congress Control Number: 2023950099

ISBN 978-1-394-21622-2 (pbk); ISBN 978-1-394-21620-8 (ebk); ISBN 978-1-394-21621-5 (ebk)

SKY10061972_120623

Contents at a Glance

Recipes at a Glance

Table of Contents

Introduction

I f you're tired of restrictive fad diets that set rigorous standards about what you can eat or make you feel guilty for enjoying certain foods, then you have come to the right place. The macro diet is your path to food freedom through nutritional empowerment.

The macro diet is an eating plan in which you track your intake of protein, carbohydrates, and fats to reach targeted intakes. On the macro diet, you get to eat meals and snacks that you enjoy and that make you feel good. You'll gain the nutritional knowledge you need to tailor a balanced and personalized program that meets *your* standards for wellness and health, not standards set by a celebrity or a social media influencer.

If you want to lose weight on this plan, you can! If you're gunning to reach a fitness goal, then the macro diet has you covered as well. Or if you simply want to feel more energized and focused throughout the day with the confidence of knowing you're fueling your body with power-packed foods, then tracking your macros is definitely for you.

The macro diet is for people who want to bolster their mental and physical well-being with evidence-based guidance. The foundations of the diet are based on hundreds of years of nutritional science, and the guidance offered aligns with the most recent recommendations provided by major health organizations based on peer-reviewed scientific studies.

So, if you're ready to take charge of your eating habits to crush your goals, then prepare yourself for a new you. The macro diet is your key to years of happy, healthy eating and enjoyment.

About This Book

This book is designed so that you have all the information you need to set up your macro diet right at your fingertips. Like all Dummies series books, you'll find that it is organized with easy access in mind.

You don't have to read the entire book or even read the chapters sequentially to design your macro diet plan. Each chapter helps you to complete a different task or master a specific skill related to macro tracking. If you are already familiar with the concepts in a particular chapter, skip it and move on to another.

However, you may want to bookmark certain pages or sections. For example, in Chapter 6, I show you how to calculate your macro targets. Since you may adjust these numbers from time to time, you might want to dog-ear those pages so you can find them easily when it's time to tweak your food plan.

You'll also want to keep in mind the following tips for the recipe chapters:

>> All temperatures are listed in degrees Fahrenheit. The appendix includes information about how to convert cooking temperatures to Celsius.

>> Eggs are always large.

>> Ground pepper is freshly ground pepper.

>> Onions are yellow (unless specified otherwise), although feel free to experiment with other varieties.

>> Recipes listed with the tomato icon are vegetarian.

>> Olive oil is extra virgin, but you can experiment with other varieties if you prefer. Extra virgin olive oil is more flavorful than regular olive oil, but it has a slightly lower smoke point than regular olive oil.

Lastly, you'll find a few web addresses listed throughout the book. If you want to visit the website, simply type the address into the address bar (at the top of your browser window) exactly as indicated without any line breaks or spaces. If you bought the digital version of this book, just click on the link to go to the web page.

Foolish Assumptions

In writing this book, I made a few assumptions about you, my reader.

>> You want to improve your health, accomplish a fitness goal, or reach or maintain a healthy weight.

>> You like the idea of gaining more energy and focus with a balanced, nutritious diet.

>> You enjoy eating, and you're tired of diet plans that tell you that you should feel guilt or shame for eating certain foods.

» You're willing to invest some time into tailoring a diet that suits your personalized needs.

» You want to gain nutritional knowledge to make food choices and meal decisions that leave you feeling empowered.

Lastly and most importantly, I assume that you are the one who knows what's best for your body, especially when it comes to your weight. The book provides information to help you reach different types of goals, including weight loss, weight maintenance, and weight gain. But I make no assumptions or recommendations about what a healthy weight is for you — that is your decision. If you are unsure of how your weight affects your health, have a conversation with your health practitioner to get personalized advice.

Icons Used in This Book

Throughout this book, icons in the margins highlight certain types of valuable information that call out for your attention. Here are the icons you'll encounter and a brief description of each.

The Tip icon marks tips and shortcuts that you can use to make following the macro diet easier.

Remember icons mark the information that's especially important to know. To siphon off the most important information in each chapter, just skim through these icons.

The Technical Stuff icon marks information of a highly technical nature that you can normally skip over.

The Warning icon tells you to watch out! It marks important information that may save you from making nutritional decisions that might compromise your physical or mental well-being.

Beyond the Book

In addition to the abundance of information and guidance related to the macro diet that I provide in this book, you get access to even more help and information online at Dummies.com. Check out this book's online Cheat Sheet. Just go to www.dummies.com and search for "Macro Diet For Dummies Cheat Sheet."

Where to Go from Here

If you are a nutrition newbie, welcome! I'm glad you're here! You might want to start with Chapter 1 and move through the book sequentially at your own pace. Remember, this isn't a short-term, quick-fix diet. Take plenty of time to grasp the underlying concepts about macros and balanced nutrition so that you appreciate the value of investing time in calculating your targets and prepping meals.

If you have a solid nutritional background, then navigate through the book as you see fit. You may want to skip Part 1 and move right into goal setting in Chapter 5. Or, if you already have a specific goal in mind for your new nutritional plan, skip Chapter 5 and get right into calculating your targets, which I explain in Chapter 6.

Regardless of where you begin, remember that the macro diet isn't a one-stop nutritional shop. You'll probably find that you want to go back and make changes from time to time. That's great! Keep the book handy so that you always have the information you need to make sure the macro diet supports you through a lifetime of wellness and vitality.

1

Getting Started with the Macro Diet

Browse the basics of the macro diet, including how it compares to other diets and whether or not to count calories.

Master nutritional basics by learning about foundational building blocks: protein, carbohydrates, and fats.

Consider macro diet benefits to see how this eating plan might affect your health and wellness goals.

Weigh the pros and cons of the macro diet to decide whether it is right for you.

Chapter **1**

Looking at the Big Picture of the Macro Diet

The macro diet is an approach to daily nutrition that helps you reach the goals that are important to *you*. It is a personalized system that allows you to reach both short- and long-term fitness, health, or weight-loss targets without the restriction required on many traditional diets.

Instead of imposing random calorie limits or eliminating certain types of food (or even entire food groups), this method allows you to build meals around the foods you enjoy — *all* of them.

If you have a type-A personality and you are a person who likes to be very specific in their eating plan, you can set up the diet so that every nutrient and calorie is measured and accounted for. You'll be satisfied knowing that you are meeting very accurate and important targets each day.

But if you prefer a more laid-back approach to eating, you can still set and reach goals on this plan to enjoy more energy and balance throughout the day.

In this chapter, I explain the most basic concepts of the diet so that you can get a bird's-eye view of the macro diet approach. I illustrate how this nutritional strategy compares to other weight-loss and diet plans so that you can make an informed choice about choosing the program. Finally, I address common questions about calories and food choices and show you how this program is grounded in well-tested nutritional science. After reading this chapter, my hope is that you will feel excited and energized about investing in a healthier new you.

Foundational Concepts of the Macro Diet

The macro diet isn't one specific nutritional prescription but rather an approach to eating that can be customized for each individual. You may notice that the diet goes by different names when people in the media refer to it.

The macro diet is sometimes called "macro tracking" or "tracking your macros." It has also been referred to as "the flexible diet" or "flexible dieting" because there are so many different ways to adapt the plan to align with your goals and lifestyle. Some people also call this the "IIFYM diet," which stands for "if it fits your macros" or "IIMYM" which stands for "if it meets your macros." All of these names refer to the same program of counting or tracking the macronutrients that you consume in the food that you eat.

REMEMBER

The word "macro" is short for macronutrient. *Macronutrients* are nutritive components of food that your body needs to function. You might think of macros as the large foundational building blocks of nutrition.

MACRO VERSUS MICRONUTRIENTS

Macronutrients are the large building blocks of nutrition. But smaller building blocks are also important. These are called "micronutrients." Micronutrients are the vitamins and minerals that your body also needs. For example, vitamin C, found in citrus fruit, is a micronutrient.

This book doesn't cover the topic of micronutrients in great detail. But if you are interested in learning more about vitamins and minerals, I go over the basics in Chapter 2, which includes a list of important micronutrients along with a list of good sources.

What is most important for you to know is that eating a balanced macronutrient diet that includes a wide range of foods, especially fruits and vegetables, can help you to get the micronutrients that you need to stay healthy.

Three macronutrients exist, and you've probably heard of them. They are protein, carbohydrate, and fat. All three macros play an important — but different — role in your body's daily processes.

>> **Protein** provides your body with amino acids to help build and repair muscle and other tissues.

>> **Carbohydrates** (also called "carbs") are your body's preferred energy source and help you to stay active and alert throughout the day.

>> **Fat** provides insulation and protection for your organs and helps to support healthy cells.

Each gram of protein, fat, or carbohydrate has a specific function. (For more detail, see Chapter 2.) Each macronutrient gram also supplies the body with calories.

Calories are simply a unit of energy. Each one of us has a different caloric requirement based on factors like body size and activity level. Because macros provide calories, when you count your macros, you could say that you are counting calories. But what makes this program different is that the macro diet puts the emphasis on the *type* of calories that you consume. The later section "Considering Calories" explains this in more detail.

REMEMBER

On the macro diet, you try to achieve specific intakes (in grams) for protein, fat, and carbohydrates rather than just counting the number of calories that you consume.

Different health and nutrition organizations provide guidelines for how much protein, fat, and carbs you should consume. But those recommendations are fairly broad. On the macro diet, you fine-tune the numbers according to your personalized needs.

The cornerstone of macro tracking is refining the percentages to get the optimal balance of protein, fat, and carbohydrate for your body. This allows you to function at your best to achieve whatever goals you've set, whether they are weight-loss goals, athletic goals, fitness goals, or general health and wellness goals.

Types of Macro Diets and Variations

A few different variations of the macro diet have become known in their own right, including the ketogenic diet and the Zone diet. You might be familiar with them. I don't detail these macro diet variations in this book simply because each one requires that you follow a specific pre-designated ratio of nutrients. In this book, I show you how to figure out your own macro balance rather than following one that is already established.

Ketogenic diet

Also known as the keto diet or "going keto," this variation of the macro diet puts the emphasis on fat consumption.

If you follow a ketogenic diet, you track your macronutrient intake, but you eat far more fat than protein or carbohydrates to put your body into a state of ketosis. Ketosis occurs when your body burns fat, rather than glucose, for fuel.

For many people, this eating plan sounds appealing because many desirable foods are high in fat, like french fries or ice cream. But many of those foods also contain high amounts of sugar or starch, which are carbohydrates. So, you're not able to eat most of the foods that you might want to eat because they prevent you from getting into or maintaining ketosis.

WARNING

On the keto diet, you consume macronutrients in proportions that fall outside of the guidelines recommended by health organizations like the U.S. Department of Health and Human Services (HHS) and the United States Department of Agriculture (USDA). So while this eating program has a history of use in medical settings, inconsistent evidence supports its use for long-term weight loss, athletic performance, or overall wellness.

The Zone diet or 40-30-30

Dr. Barry Sears developed this eating plan that became popular in the 1990s. It is an eating plan based on counting macronutrients rather than counting calories. The diet has maintained a significant following since the '90s and is now sold as a commercial diet plan. But many people use general zone principles as the basis for an eating program rather than signing up for the commercial plan.

On the Zone diet, you consume a 40-30-30 macro balance where 40 percent of your calories come from carbohydrates (like colorful veggies and fruit), 30 percent of your calories come from lean proteins (think fish, lean beef, or poultry), and 30 percent comes from healthy fats such as nuts, olive oil, or avocado.

TIP

The Zone diet differs from the macro diet described in this book because everyone on the Zone follows the same macro ratio. Whereas in this book, I show you how to base your ratios on your own personal needs.

IS THE MACRO DIET THE SAME AS THE MACROBIOTIC DIET?

Even though their names are similar, the macro diet and the macrobiotic diet are two different programs. The macro diet is based on the fact that you need to consume a balanced diet of three macronutrients. You tailor those macros to meet your own personalized needs.

On the macrobiotic diet you consume unprocessed organic foods. You avoid foods that are high in fat, processed, salty, or sugary, including dairy, meat, and eggs. Fans of the diet believe that this helps to achieve balance and harmony while removing toxins from the body.

The macrobiotic diet is considered to be a very stringent diet. The list of non-compliant foods is fairly substantial. On the macro diet, you'll have much more leeway to make food choices that align with your goals.

While the Zone diet remains popular, it falls (slightly) short compared to recommended nutrition guidelines. USDA guidelines suggest that you consume at least 45 percent of your total daily calories from carbohydrates, whereas on this plan, you consume only 40 percent of your daily calories from carbs. For that reason, some people find this eating plan hard to maintain.

Plant-based macro diets

A plant-based diet isn't necessarily a macro diet, but it can be. There are different types of plant-based eating, and you can use macro tracking with any of them.

>> **Plant-based** eating is a diet on which most of the foods you consume come from plants. But you may occasionally consume meat, dairy, or seafood as no foods are technically "off-limits."

>> **Vegetarian** diets are those that eliminate any animal-based food, but might include eggs and dairy.

>> **Vegan** diets are those that eliminate all animal-based products, including eggs, dairy, and foods like honey or gelatin (when it is made with animal collagen).

Many macro trackers focus on getting enough protein in their diets. They build meals specifically to make sure that they reach their protein targets. Since protein often comes from animal products, you might be surprised that you can follow the macro diet even if you eat only plant-based foods.

TIP

This book provides plenty of resources, including food lists and recipes, that can help you to follow a plant-based macro diet.

Seeing How the Macro Diet Differs from Other Diets

To help you understand what the macro diet *is*, it may be helpful to show you what it *isn't*. Here's how macro tracking compares to popular eating plans you may be familiar with.

Restrictive, commercial, and elimination diets

Commercial diets, like Weight Watchers, Jenny Craig, Nutrisystem, and others, often require you to sign up and pay for a service that may include coaching from others who have been successful on the plan and food delivery services.

To be successful on these plans, you often rely on portion-controlled pre-made entrees and snacks. Sometimes, you must eliminate or significantly reduce your intake of certain foods or food groups. For example, during the early weeks of the Atkins diet, you significantly restrict your intake of carbohydrates.

On the macro diet, however, you're the one in the driver's seat. This is not a commercial plan; there is no company to pay or service to sign up for. You decide what foods to consume and what foods to cut back on.

Food delivery companies may provide macro-balanced meals for a fee, but you don't have to sign up for any food delivery service to follow this plan. In fact, most people do their own food and meal prep. In Chapter 8, I show you how to set up your kitchen and prep meals like a pro. In Part 5, you'll find recipes for everything from smoothies to satisfying entrees and even desserts and snacks.

Whole 30, Mediterranean, and Paleo

When you follow a diet like the Whole 30 diet, the Mediterranean diet, or the Paleo diet, you choose foods or avoid foods based on the characteristics of the food rather than on a product's nutritional makeup.

For instance, on the Whole 30 diet, you eliminate most processed foods (such as those that include added sugar, artificial sugar alternatives, and other additives) for a period of 30 days. On the Paleo diet, you consume only foods that would have been eaten during the Paleolithic era. On the Mediterranean diet, you choose foods that are typically consumed in the Mediterranean region, especially Greece.

REMEMBER

On the macro diet, it doesn't matter where your food comes from or how it is processed. You choose foods and build meals solely based on nutritional makeup.

If the theories behind Whole30, the Mediterranean diet, or the Paleo diet appeal to you, you can still follow the macro diet and choose foods that align with those eating plans as well.

Intermittent fasting

Intermittent fasting is a time-restricted eating plan. In some ways, it is similar to the macro diet because no foods are required or off-limits. But the thinking behind the diet is very different.

When you practice intermittent fasting, you can eat anything you want if you limit your food intake to a specific time window. The goal is to reduce or limit total caloric intake by reducing the time you spend eating during the day.

For instance, some people follow a 18/6 intermittent fasting plan in which they fast for 18 hours and limit their food intake to six hours during the day. Other popular plans include the 12/12 plan and the 14/10 plan.

On the macro diet, timing doesn't matter (unless you want it to). I discuss nutrient timing in Chapter 8, but you do not have to follow any specific guidelines about *when* to eat. The focus on the macro diet is reaching nutritional targets rather than limiting food intake.

Considering Calories

When it comes to diets — commercial diets, popular diets, or wholistic diets — calories are usually a primary consideration. After all, people often adopt a new eating plan to change their body weight. And calories matter when weight loss or weight gain is the goal.

Many people (myself included!) believe that tracking macros is healthier than counting calories. But the relationship between macros and calories is tricky. Here's why: If you are counting macros, you *are* counting calories. So, to say that one is healthier than the other can be confusing and a bit contradictory. In this section, I dive into this idea a little bit deeper so you can understand the relationship between counting calories and counting macros.

Calories are simply a unit of energy. A calorie is a unit of heat equivalent to the energy needed to raise the temperature of one gram of water by one degree Celsius.

Your body uses energy — from calories — for fuel. You need calories to maintain basic functions like blood circulation and breathing and for other activities, including exercise and non-exercise movement.

The number of calories you need depends on factors including your body size (height and weight), your sex, your age, and your activity level. But most adults have a calorie requirement that falls within a certain range.

According to the 2020–2025 Dietary Guidelines for Americans, adult women need roughly 1,600 calories to 2,400 calories per day, and men need about 2,200 to 3,200 calories per day. These numbers are in line with numbers provided by peer-reviewed nutritional studies and consistent with suggestions provided by the World Health Organization.

You can figure out how many calories you burn each day to determine your personalized calorie needs. Chapter 6 explains how to calculate your number. For now, it is just important to understand that calories provide energy and each macronutrient supplies a different amount.

Carbohydrates and protein each supply your body with four calories of energy per gram. Fat supplies your body with nine calories of energy per gram.

So, if you understand that macronutrients supply your body with calories, you can see why counting macros can be considered a variation of counting calories. But counting macros doesn't necessarily mean you should disregard the generalized concept of caloric intake.

A successful macro tracking plan can — and in many cases should — still take total caloric intake into account, especially if weight loss or weight gain is your goal.

Why calories (still) matter

Most of us don't have a very good idea of the number of calories we consume each day. In fact, several research studies have suggested that we have a tendency to underestimate our caloric intake. But if you eat when you're hungry and stop eating when you're full, you're likely to consume the number of calories that your body needs. But you and I both know that we often eat — or overeat — for reasons other than hunger.

So, what happens if you consume more calories than you need? It doesn't matter if those extra calories come from fat, carbohydrate, or protein; your body will store the extra energy to use later. Over time, an energy surplus can lead to weight gain.

TIP

Weight gain occurs when you consume more energy — or calories — than you need. Your body stores the extra energy as fat.

Unfortunately, you can't decide where your body will store those excess calories. Some people store fat in their midsection, while others store it on their hips and thighs.

Over time, fat is likely to accumulate all over your body if you continue to consume excess calories. The fat stores will remain until your body needs those extra calories for energy. This occurs when you consume fewer calories than you need, creating a calorie deficit. A calorie deficit causes you to lose weight.

REMEMBER

Even if you count your macros and consume a healthy, balanced ratio of protein, fat, and carbohydrates, you won't lose weight until a sustained calorie deficit exists.

To ensure you are creating a calorie deficit each day, it's probably best to count those calories. So, how much of a calorie deficit do you need to slim down? The exact number is a topic of great debate. Most experts agree that a pound of fat is roughly equivalent to about 3,500 calories. So, to lose a pound of fat, you should create a deficit of approximately 3,500 calories.

To slim down safely, you'll want to accomplish the 3,500-calorie deficit over time. For instance, to create a weekly deficit of 3,500 calories and lose one pound per week (considered a safe rate of weight loss), you could create a daily calorie deficit of 500 calories.

500 calories × 7 days = 3,500 calories or about one pound of fat

In short, calories still matter when you are tracking macros — especially when weight loss is your primary target. In Chapter 6, I show you exactly how to create a calorie deficit for weight loss if that is your goal.

But here is where tracking your macros hits a home run. Getting a balance of macronutrients can help to curb hunger, help you to stay energized throughout the day, and help you to feel full and satisfied after eating. You're more likely to consume the right number of calories if your body is supplied with a healthy balance of nutrients.

But that's not all! Counting macros can be more beneficial for your body than just counting calories, whether weight loss is your goal or not.

The benefits of counting macros versus counting calories

While calories matter — especially for weight loss, counting your macros is more advantageous than simply counting calories. Consider these benefits.

Tracking macros takes nutritional value into account

When you count calories, there isn't necessarily an incentive to choose healthy foods or improve the quality of your diet or overall wellness. The quantity of the calories matters, but quality isn't part of the equation.

When you track macros, on the other hand, you ensure that you get a nutritious balance of protein, fat, and carbohydrates. Each macro plays a role in supporting good health.

Tracking macros allows for greater customization

If you are trying to lose (or gain) weight, you can use your activity level and other factors to calculate your caloric needs. But the number you get doesn't necessarily consider your current body composition or any body composition goals. It also doesn't take into account any athletic goals.

For instance, if you want to maintain or gain muscle, you'll want a higher percentage of calories to come from protein. And if you are a runner, cyclist, or participate in long cardio workouts, you'll want a significant percentage of calories to come from carbohydrates.

Macro tracking allows you to use a calorie target to reach your desired weight, but it also helps to support your training and body composition goals as well.

Macro tracking promotes abundance rather than restriction

Cutting calories can feel restrictive, especially if you've set a low or very low calorie goal (which is never recommended except under a physician's guidance). The focus is often on eating less and cutting back. In some cases, you may even eliminate certain foods from your diet because they are high in fat or calories.

When you track macros, you are encouraged to eat foods that you enjoy to reach your targets. In fact, you may even find yourself adding foods to your meal plan to ensure you get enough fat, protein, or carbohydrate.

TIP

When you shift your mental focus to "filling up" rather than "cutting back," making dietary changes becomes mentally easier to manage.

Answering the Big Question: Can I Really Eat Anything I Want?

The macro diet is often called the flexible diet because you are the one in the driver's seat when it comes to food choices.

REMEMBER

No "good" foods or "bad" foods are on the macro diet, and no food or type of food is off-limits. In fact, the more you build your meals around foods you enjoy, the more likely you are to stick with your plan and reach your goals.

That's why, when you scroll through social media channels, you often see images of pizza, brownies, burgers (and other foods that aren't typically associated with healthy eating) tagged with the IIFYM hashtag. The belief is that "if it meets your macros," you can eat whatever you want. So, you can enjoy that burger and milk-shake or cheesy slice of pizza as long as you meet your targets for each macro at the end of the day.

Eating a diet without limitations comes with pros and cons. *Can* you eat whatever you want on the macro diet? Yes. But you may not always want to, depending on your goals.

As you stock your fridge and fill your pantry with macro-balanced foods, consider the pros and cons of limitless eating versus a more mindful or intuitive approach to eating, in which you balance indulgent foods with nutrient-rich, less processed foods.

The case for limitless eating

If you are a person who currently consumes a standard American diet, shifting immediately to a diet that includes primarily fruits, veggies, lean proteins, and plant-based fats may not be realistic.

TECHNICAL STUFF

The standard American diet, sometimes called the SAD diet, is the diet of many Americans. It consists primarily of ultra-processed foods, added sugar, fat, and sodium.

If you consume this type of diet, you may visit fast food restaurants regularly. You might have a freezer full of manufactured, heavily processed meals. This diet is generally lacking in fresh fruits and vegetables, legumes, whole grains, healthy fats, and lean protein.

When you eat foods with excess salt and sugar, the way you taste food changes. You are more likely to crave ultra-processed foods because that is what your palate is used to. Changing that habit might be challenging. Eating wholesome foods with more subtle flavors may not feel satisfying — even if they are more nutritious.

For example, if you meet your carb intake target with fruits and vegetables, your body will likely feel better over time than if you meet that target with sugary sodas and processed, starchy, high-sodium snacks. But if you really enjoy those snacks and beverages, you won't feel good about giving them up.

TIP

If you currently consume a SAD diet, the smartest approach initially will be to make small, gradual adjustments. Your initial goal for the macro diet may simply be to consume a more balanced diet to enjoy the benefits of better nutrition. You don't want to set any other limits on your food choices at this stage to keep the diet sustainable.

So, in the beginning, you might choose those processed foods that you enjoy and that you are familiar with. You'll focus on ensuring you get adequate amounts of each macro at this stage.

Then, as you feel more comfortable reaching macro targets, you can set a goal to improve diet quality. At that point, you can add foods like fruits and veggies or whole grains. As you find healthy foods you enjoy, you might find that setting limits on less healthy processed foods feels good.

The point here is that every dieter will have their own unique starting point. To keep this diet healthy, you need to make small gradual adjustments and always include foods that you love. Enjoying your meals is an important part of what makes the macro diet healthy and sustainable.

The case against limitless eating

Some people use the macro diet to support substantial (and sometimes even aggressive) athletic training or body composition goals. In most cases, these people already have a fairly stringent workout and nutritional plan in place. If you're one of these people, you are probably already familiar with making sacrifices to achieve your goals.

TIP

If you have set high expectations for reaching certain training, performance, or body composition goals, you'll have less room to include indulgent foods in your macro diet. In this situation, every calorie needs to provide the highest quality fuel to support your workouts and/or competitive events.

Of course, that doesn't mean you can't enjoy an indulgent meal or a treat from time to time, but the bottom line is that if you set the bar high for your fitness endeavors, your diet will also need to rise to those standards.

How (and why) to find a happy medium

The cases for and against limitless eating describe two ends of the nutritional spectrum. Most people who read this book will fall somewhere in the middle.

Maybe you are a person who includes wholesome foods in your diet along with occasional fast-food goodies and indulgent treats. And maybe you'd like to lose a little fat, gain a little muscle, and improve your cardiovascular endurance slightly, but you're not interested in doing fitness competitions or spending your life at the gym.

There are ways to find a happy medium between eating everything you want and restricting yourself to a stringent macro diet.

TIP

By learning to listen to your body and practice mindful eating, you can include the foods you love on the macro diet and still reach fitness and health goals.

So how does that look on a day-to-day basis? It simply means that you become mindful of your body's needs and make informed choices about meeting them.

For example, let's say that you've set up your macro diet, and it includes a hearty breakfast that you enjoy but leaves you hungry and craving carbs in the late morning hours. Out of habit, you always head to the vending machine in your office building and grab a processed sugary snack. It doesn't align with your macro plan, but it gives you the boost you need to get on with your day until lunchtime.

A healthier approach to this scenario might include some pre-planning and adaptation. If you notice that you get hungry a few hours after breakfast, then you might want to make adjustments. Include more calories in your morning meal or add some high-fiber whole grains to help you to feel fuller longer after eating. You could also pack a healthy snack (see Chapter 17) or smoothie (see Chapter 14). This might eliminate the cravings altogether.

But what if you really look forward to that vending machine treat? If that is the case, you should keep it in your diet and include the calories in your macro plan. There is nothing wrong with enjoying your vending machine goodie! But it should be a mindful decision, and eating it should be an enjoyable occasion. Just grabbing the snack out of habit isn't doing you any favors.

When you start to listen to your body and make mindful choices, you're likely to find a happy balance where you give your body the nutrition it needs, but you also treat yourself to foods that you love simply because they are enjoyable to eat.

You can build your macro plan to include any food, but it will probably require you to make choices here and there about what to include in your meal and what to skip. But sometimes making those choices helps you to enjoy food more fully.

Deciding If It's Just a Fad

If you scroll through social media channels, you'll probably notice that IIFYM and macro tracking are well-established trends. But is the macro diet really a fad?

For hundreds of years, nutritional researchers have understood the importance of protein, fat, and carbohydrates as key components of our diet. Building our diets around a balance of these nutrients gained traction after World War II. But the way that a macro-based diet has been marketed recently has vaulted its popularity in the media, making it look like a temporary diet craze.

Celebrities like Carrie Underwood, Hilary Duff, The Rock, and Chris Hemsworth have all been associated with the macro diet. Celebrity trainers also mention the diet regularly when they talk about the nutritional advice that they give to the stars. And there is no shortage of social media influencers (#fitfluencers) who share images of meals that align with their macro tracking program. But you shouldn't follow this program because your favorite celeb or Instagram personality brags about it. You should follow it because it feels right for you.

Every five years the U. S. Department of Agriculture provides recommendations regarding the proportion of calories that you should consume from protein, fat, and carbs. These guidelines date back to the late 1890s. So, this eating style has stood the test of time.

Nutritional experts throughout the years have repeatedly advised that consuming a balanced diet is important for good health. Countless research studies have also acknowledged the importance of consuming a range of nutrients and a wide range of foods.

The macro diet helps you to learn more about the macronutrient balance that your body needs and how much better your body works when you give it the nutrition it needs. The basic principles of the macro diet are not likely to change. It doesn't matter what label you use, balanced nutrition is here to stay.

Chapter **2**

Understanding the Building Blocks: Macronutrients

Six nutrients allow your body to function at its best: protein, fat, carbohydrates, vitamins, minerals, and water. On the macro diet, you'll concern yourself primarily with the three macronutrients: protein, carbohydrates, and fat. Vitamins, minerals, and water are no less important, and I also tell you how to ensure adequate intakes of each, but your day-to-day tracking will concern macros.

The calories in protein, carbohydrates, and fat all provide your body with energy. In addition to supplying energy, each macronutrient serves other bodily functions.

The more you can understand these functions, the more motivated you may become to make sure you get enough of each nutrient.

TIP

Understanding each nutrient's role may also help you to determine the best macro balance for you. For instance, if your primary goal is to build muscle, you probably want to prioritize protein intake.

In this chapter, I detail the function of each macronutrient and compare different types of food that provide these nutrients. I also touch on the role of micronutrients — vitamins and minerals — and explain how to reach the recommended daily allowance for each one. Finally, I tell you about how hydration matters throughout the day and how to make sure that you get enough water to stay healthy and energized.

What Is Protein?

When most people think of protein, they think of meat. Foods like beef, poultry, pork, and game meats are certainly good sources of protein. But there are many other sources to choose from as well. So, if you are not a meat eater or if you prefer to consume less meat for ethical or environmental reasons, you can find many other protein-rich foods to consume.

But first, let's take a step back and learn why protein is important for a strong and healthy body.

What protein does in the body

Protein is sometimes called the "building block of life" because it helps to build and repair cells. It provides structure and form to hair, skin, nails, muscle, bone, and other tissues. Protein also promotes healthy immune function and helps deliver oxygen to our cells. We need protein throughout our lives, but especially when we are young.

TIP

Protein is important during all stages of life but especially in the early stages when we are growing rapidly.

Protein is made up of long chains of amino acids. Amino acids are molecules that can be combined in different ways to make different types of protein to serve different functions.

Twenty different types of amino acids exist. Your body makes most of them, but nine are considered essential amino acids because your body doesn't make them. You must consume essential amino acids in the food that you eat.

TECHNICAL STUFF

Some amino acids are called branched-chain amino acids (BCAAs) because of their particular structure. These three amino acids are believed to be especially important for stimulating muscle protein synthesis or muscle building, among other functions.

The nine essential amino acids are

>> **Histidine:** A brain chemical that helps support digestion, a healthy immune system, proper sleep, and sexual function.

>> **Isoleucine:** A branched-chain amino acid that helps to make hemoglobin and is needed for muscle metabolism.

>> **Leucine:** A branched-chain amino acid that helps to build and repair muscles, heal wounds, and regulate blood sugar levels. Leucine may also increase the production of human growth hormone.

>> **Lysine:** A compound also called L-lysine, involved in hormone production and important for calcium absorption and immune function.

>> **Methionine:** An amino acid that contains sulfur and is important for proper growth and development, metabolism, and the absorption of certain minerals.

>> **Phenylalanine:** A compound that helps to produce other amino acids and may help to improve mood, alertness, learning, and memory.

>> **Threonine:** An amino acid important for normal blood clotting, and healthy skin and connective tissue. It is also essential for gut health and plays a role in fat metabolism.

>> **Tryptophan:** A commonly known amino acid that helps to make serotonin, a brain chemical that helps to regulate mood, appetite, and sleep.

>> **Valine:** A branched-chain amino acid involved in muscle growth, tissue regeneration, and energy production.

When you consume protein in foods such as meat, fish, soy, dairy, nuts, whole grains, and certain vegetables, you should get the amino acids you need. However, you'll still see many supplements on the market that contain amino acids, especially branched-chain amino acids.

For general health, nutrition experts usually recommend getting your protein from whole foods rather than supplements. However, the International Society of Sports Nutrition (ISSN) acknowledges that in some cases, supplements may be the most efficient way for athletes to get the amino acids that they need, especially branched-chain amino acids.

In Chapter 6, I go into more detail about the protein needs of athletes, both strength-trained athletes (weightlifters) and endurance athletes (runners, swimmers, cyclists). In that chapter, you can compare your training volume to guidelines offered by sports nutrition organizations. Then you'll be able to calculate your exact protein needs.

But guidelines offered by sports organizations generally align with the recommendations provided by general health organizations for overall wellness. These organizations include the U.S. Department of Health and Human Services and the U.S. Department of Agriculture, the two organizations that publish dietary guidelines for Americans every five years.

REMEMBER

The Dietary Guidelines for Americans advise that you consume between 10 percent and 35 percent of your daily calories from protein.

That means if you consume 2,000 calories per day, you'd aim to get 200 to 700 calories from protein (50–175 grams). If you consume 1,800 calories per day, you'd shoot for 45–158 grams of protein per day, and if you consume 2,500 calories per day, you'd try to get 63–219 grams of protein per day.

Different types of protein

Protein is often associated with meat. But you can select from many other sources of protein as well, including plant and nonmeat animal-based foods.

If you're an omnivore (you eat all types of food) you'll do your body a favor by consuming both plant- and animal-based protein foods to get a wide range of nutrients. But if you are a vegan or vegetarian, you'll want to familiarize yourself with plant-based sources.

In Chapter 8, you'll find a list of protein foods organized by the grocery store section. That list contains both animal- and plant-based foods. Use that list when you shop for protein foods.

Animal-based protein

When people think of protein, they often think of meat. Common animal protein sources include beef, chicken, turkey, seafood, eggs, and dairy products.

Protein supplements, like protein powder, are also commonly used to increase protein intake. Protein powders may be made from plant sources (like soy) or animal sources (like whey, a component of milk).

Animal-based protein sources are often believed to have better muscle-building properties than plant-based protein foods. However, some studies have challenged that belief.

For instance, a 2021 large-scale research review published in the journal *Nutrients* found that both plant and animal protein sources helped improve overall muscular strength in people of all ages. But they did find that animal protein had a slight edge over plant-based protein when it came to the percentage of lean muscle mass, especially in younger adults.

One of the reasons that animal protein is sometimes preferred is because animal proteins are sources of complete proteins. *Complete proteins* are those protein foods that contain all nine essential amino acids.

So, when you consume protein from animal sources, you know you're giving your body all of those amino acids that it can't make on its own. But you might be giving your body some other nutrients that you may want to limit.

WARNING

Animal-based proteins are also likely to contain saturated fat, which is linked to heart disease and other conditions. Some studies have linked red meat consumption to an increased risk of heart disease, stroke, and early death. But those findings are controversial, as is the role saturated fat plays in overall health.

I cover the controversy about saturated fat in the section "Different types of fat" later in this chapter. Still, if you have been told to limit your intake, then you may want to stick to those animal-based protein choices that contain less saturated fat, such as lean poultry and seafood. You might also want to consider filling up on plant-based protein.

Plant-based protein

Many people choose plant-based protein over animal protein because they believe it to be superior for overall heart health and increased longevity. Some studies have supported this argument.

A widely cited, large-scale review published in a 2021 issue of *JAMA Internal Medicine* found that substituting animal protein with plant protein was associated with a lower risk of all-cause mortality (death from any cause), death from cardiovascular disease, and death from dementia. The study authors also found that consuming nuts instead of red meat, eggs, or dairy was associated with a lower risk of death from any cause.

Scientific findings like these have convinced many people to eliminate animal proteins from their diet completely or significantly reduce their intake in favor of plant-based protein.

TIP

Popular plant-based proteins include foods like soy, some whole grains (like quinoa), beans, legumes, nuts, seeds, and certain leafy greens, like spinach and kale.

However, you should consider two primary trade-offs when you swap out animal products for plant products.

REMEMBER

Plant-based sources usually contain less protein than animal products. So, you may have to eat more plant-based foods to meet your protein needs. Second, most plant-based proteins are not complete proteins.

A few plant-based foods are complete proteins. These include quinoa, soy, chia seeds, buckwheat, and a few others. You can also combine foods, like rice and beans, to get all of the amino acids that you need. Foods that work together to provide you with all of the essential amino acids are called *complementary proteins*. And you don't need to consume those complementary proteins in the same meal. Just make sure you incorporate them in your diet throughout the day.

Another benefit of plant-based protein is that these foods are generally lower in fat and calories than animal sources. If your goal is weight loss, you can keep your caloric intake within your target range more easily with plant-based proteins than with foods like hamburger or dairy products.

People choose plant-based protein sources over animal-based sources for many other reasons. Some people do so for ethical reasons (to support animal rights), and others do it for environmental reasons.

From a nutritional standpoint, both plant- and animal-based proteins can help you to reach your intake needs. So, choose the foods that align with your beliefs and your food preferences.

What Are Carbohydrates?

Carbohydrates are your body's preferred energy source. For this reason, nutrition experts recommend that the largest proportion of our calories come from carbs (as opposed to fat or protein).

REMEMBER

According to the Dietary Guidelines for Americans, 45 percent to 65 percent of your calories should come from carbohydrates.

So, if you consume 2,000 calories per day, you'd aim to get 900 to 1,300 calories from carbs or 225–325 grams. If you consume 1,800 calories per day, you'd shoot for 203–293 grams of carbohydrates per day, and if you consume 2,500 calories per day, you'd try to get 281–406 grams of carbohydrates per day.

Unfortunately, this macronutrient has gotten a bad reputation in recent years because some people believe that carbs make you gain weight or that carbs are unhealthy. Neither statement is true.

Carbs aren't "good" or "bad," but some carbohydrates provide better nutrition than others. Carbohydrates, when consumed in excess, can contribute to weight gain, just like protein and fat.

Understanding what carbs do in the body and the different types of carbs can help you to make the best decision about which carbs are best for you, depending on your situation.

What carbs do in the body

Carbohydrates provide energy to the body. Fat and protein can also supply energy, but your body prefers carbohydrates because they are broken down with the least amount of effort.

Carbohydrates are classified according to their chemical structure. Carbs can be simple or complex.

>> **Simple carbohydrates** are those that contain one or two sugar molecules. They can be broken down easily in the body to provide quick energy. For example, glucose, fructose, and galactose are simple carbs that contain just one sugar molecule (monosaccharides). Table sugar (sucrose) and lactose (the sugar found naturally in milk) contain two sugar molecules (disaccharides).

>> **Complex carbohydrates** are those that have a more complicated chemical structure. They require a little more work to break down in the body.

Carbohydrate digestion begins in the mouth and continues in the digestive system (primarily in the small intestine), where complex and simple carbs combine with enzymes and are broken down into glucose, a monosaccharide.

Glucose (blood sugar) is absorbed into the bloodstream to be used as energy with the help of a hormone called insulin. If glucose isn't used as energy, it can be stored in the muscles, liver, or as *adipose tissue* (fat).

TECHNICAL STUFF

If you have too much glucose in your bloodstream, it is called *hyperglycemia* (a condition common in people with diabetes). Hyperglycemia can cause symptoms like increased thirst, needing to urinate frequently, hunger, or fatigue. Too little blood sugar is referred to as hypoglycemia.

WHAT IS THE GLYCEMIC INDEX?

The *glycemic index* is a rating system that measures how quickly or slowly carbohydrates are turned into blood glucose. Foods that are high on the glycemic index are those that turn into glucose quickly and lead to a blood sugar spike. Often, these spikes are followed by dips in blood sugar, sometimes referred to as a "sugar crash." Foods that are low on the glycemic index are those that enter the bloodstream slowly and provide a steady stream of energy.

Foods that are high on the glycemic index include foods like table sugar, honey, white rice, and processed sugary cereals. Foods that are low on the glycemic index are foods that contain fiber, like whole grains, vegetables, some fruits, and legumes.

You can find the glycemic index of a food by checking the Glycemic Index Database maintained online by the University of Sydney (Australia). Some weight-loss and nutrition experts believe that choosing foods that are lower on the glycemic index can be helpful in weight control. Studies investigating the glycemic index for weight loss have yielded mixed results.

Different types of carbs

Simple and complex carbohydrates can come in different forms, including sugars, starches, and fiber.

>> **Sugars** are simple carbohydrates (also called simple sugars). Simple sugars can occur naturally in some foods, like in fruit (fructose) or in milk (lactose). Table sugar (sucrose) is also a simple sugar. But simple sugars might also be added to foods such as candy, sodas, and other sweetened beverages, baked goods, or even in foods where you wouldn't expect to find sugar, like soups, peanut butter, or ketchup. These would be listed as "Added sugar" on the Nutrition Facts label.

>> **Starches** are complex carbohydrates. Starch is naturally found in plants, so many grains and vegetables are starchy carbs. For example, potatoes, rice, and peas are starchy carbohydrates.

>> **Fiber** is a complex carbohydrate that also comes from plants. Unlike other carbohydrates, your body can't digest fiber, so it passes through your digestive system without being broken down. Food can contain two types of fiber, soluble and insoluble. Soluble fiber dissolves and turns to gel when it mixes with water in the digestive tract. Insoluble fiber does not dissolve in water, and it passes through your digestive tract adding bulk to your stool.

COUNTING NET CARBS VERSUS TOTAL CARBS

You may hear people talking about counting "net carbs" rather than total carbohydrate grams when tracking their macros. You might also see the number of net carbs in a food advertised on the package.

Net carbs refers to the number of total carbs minus the amount of fiber and sugar alcohols in a food. Sugar alcohols are non-caloric food ingredients used as sweeteners or bulking agents.

Since fiber is not digested in the body, it does not contribute calories the way other nutrients do. Therefore, some people don't count those grams in their tracking endeavors.

The problem with counting net carbs rather than carbs is that researchers don't know exactly how many (if any) calories are provided by fiber. The U.S. Food and Drug Administration (FDA) has estimated that soluble fiber contains about two calories per gram, while insoluble fiber provides no calories at all.

The American Diabetes Association and the FDA recommend counting total carbs rather than net carbs. Even though you may see "net carbs" mentioned on some food packages, the term has no legal definition.

A food may contain more than one type of carbohydrate. For example, an apple contains sugar (fructose) and fiber. Black beans contain fiber and starch.

When choosing foods for your snacks and meals, each type of carbohydrate can contribute to a healthy diet. Foods that contain simple sugars, like fruit juice, milk, yogurt, or honey can provide a quick burst of energy. This might be helpful before a workout. Foods that contain starch might also be helpful if you need energy quickly.

TIP

Food that contains fiber is best when you need a steady stream of energy. Since it is broken down slowly, fiber helps you to feel full longer after eating, which can be especially helpful if you are trying to lose weight.

Fiber also provides other health benefits. For instance, consuming a fiber-rich diet has been associated with a lower risk for heart disease, diabetes, diverticulitis, inflammatory bowel syndrome, obesity, and colorectal cancer.

The Dietary Guidelines for Americans suggests that women consume 22-28 grams of fiber per day and that men consume 28-34 grams of fiber per day. Other countries provide similar suggestions. The European Food Safety Authority recommends an intake of 25 grams of fiber per day for adults and the Canadian government suggests that women consume 25 grams of fiber today and men consume 38 grams per day.

Unfortunately, most of us don't consume nearly enough fiber. You'll get fiber from foods like fresh fruits and vegetables, beans, and legumes. If you buy packaged foods, you can check the Nutrition Facts label to see how much fiber the food provides. Fiber is listed under Carbohydrates.

To get more fiber in your diet, you'll also want to swap out refined or enriched grains for whole grains. Foods that contain enriched or refined grains have been processed to remove the part of the grain that provides fiber.

Check out Chapter 8 to see where you'll find healthy carbohydrate foods in the grocery store. Remember, the less processed a food is, the better it will be for your body. Look for foods that are in their most natural form to maximize nutrition and health benefits for your body.

What Is Fat?

Dietary fat is the fat you consume in food, like butter or olive oil. It is different from the fat on your body, called adipose tissue. The fat on your body is either subcutaneous fat (under the skin) or visceral fat (around the organs). Subcutaneous fat and visceral help protect your organs and provide insulation.

When you consume fat in food, it doesn't necessarily turn into fat stored on your body. Any excess calories can be stored as adipose tissue or body fat.

In this section, I tell you about dietary fat. Dietary fat plays several important roles in the body, so it is important to consume enough of it and to make healthy choices when consuming fatty foods.

The Dietary Guidelines for Americans suggest that adult men and women consume between 20 percent and 35 percent of their daily calories from fat.

Fat is much more calorie-dense than carbs or protein. Protein and carbohydrates each provide four calories per gram. Fat on the other hand, provides nine calories per gram. You have to consume far less fat to meet your recommended intake.

If you consume 2,000 calories per day, you'd aim to get 400 to 700 calories from fat or 44–77 grams. If you consume 1,800 calories per day, you'd shoot for 40–70 grams of fat per day, and if you consume 2,500 calories per day, you'd try to get 55–97 grams of fat per day.

Learning more about the different types of fat and the important roles that it plays in your body can help you to choose and consume the healthiest fatty foods while on the macro diet.

What fat does in the body

One of fat's primary jobs is to supply energy to the body. Carbs are still the body's preferred energy source, but fat is packed with calories, so after carbs are expended, fat is a ready supply of energy.

But fat has other functions as well. Your body needs fat to maintain healthy cells. Cell membranes are made up (partially) of fat, so you need fat to grow and remain healthy.

Other bodily functions, such as blood clotting, nervous system function, reproduction, and immune response, are also dependent on fat to work properly. And fat plays an important role in maintaining healthy skin and nails. Some vitamins, specifically A, D, E, and K, are fat-soluble. That means you need fat to absorb those important micronutrients and use them in the body. And surprisingly, if weight loss is your goal on the macro diet, fat is especially important for you.

Fat provides a flavor and mouth feel that is satisfying and enjoyable. Simply put, fat tastes good and helps make food taste delicious so eating is enjoyable. The (failed) low-fat diet craze taught us that cutting out fat generally backfires. We usually replace fat with other less healthy ingredients, like sugar.

TIP

It's best to keep fat in your diet if you are trying to slim down. But you can make healthy fat choices and keep your intake moderate.

Different types of fat

Fat is found in almost all animal products. But there are also a wide range of plant-based fats. Fat can be divided into three main categories:

>> **Saturated fats** are generally solid at room temperature and come from animal sources. Butter, for example, is a saturated fat, and so is lard. You'll also consume saturated fat when you eat beef, pork, or other fatty meats. Many processed and fast foods contain saturated fat.

>> **Unsaturated fat** is generally liquid at room temperature and can come from plant or seafood sources. Olive oil is an unsaturated fat as is the fat in avocados. And most of the fat in seafood, like tuna and salmon, is unsaturated.

>> **Trans fats** can be natural or artificial. Dairy products, beef, and lamb contain small amounts of naturally formed trans fats. Artificial trans fats are partially hydrogenated oils found in many packaged baked goods and other highly processed foods.

These have been banned by the FDA so you should not find them in most foods purchased in the United States, but you will still see a listing for Trans Fat on the Nutrition Facts label.

REMEMBER

The 2020–2025 Dietary Guidelines for Americans still advises that you limit your intake of saturated fat to no more than 10 percent of your total daily calories.

That means if you consume a 2,000-calorie per day diet, you should consume no more than 200 calories or 22 grams of saturated fat. If you consume 1,800 calories per day, keep your saturated fat grams below 20 grams, and if you consume 2,500 calories per day, keep it under 28 grams.

ARE SATURATED FATS REALLY BAD?

Saturated fats are often identified as "bad" fats, while unsaturated fats are often identified as "good" fats. However, there is some disagreement in the nutrition and health community about whether or not saturated fat is really bad for your body.

Beginning in the 1950s, researchers began to associate the intake of saturated fat with heart disease. The idea became known as the "diet-heart hypothesis." It was based on the belief that saturated fat raises blood cholesterol, and high cholesterol puts you at higher risk for heart disease.

Some recent studies, however, have challenged the notion that saturated fat is linked to cardiovascular disease, cardiovascular mortality, or total mortality (death from any cause). But there is a lack of agreement among experts about whether or not saturated fat does or does not increase your risk for heart problems and other diseases.

If you're unsure about your intake of saturated fat, talk to your healthcare provider. They can evaluate your health history and make personalized suggestions.

As a basis for reference, a sirloin steak (160 grams or about 5.5 ounces) contains about 27 grams of total fat and about 10.5 grams of saturated fat. If you pair that with a baked potato topped with two tablespoons of butter (14g saturated fat) and two tablespoons of sour cream (2.5 grams saturated fat), your saturated fat intake would be about 27 grams.

WARNING

Fat is calorie-dense, so a small amount adds up quickly. If you are unsure about whether or not you should be concerned about your saturated fat intake, talk to your healthcare provider. Together you can evaluate your health history and your risk for heart disease and make the best decision for you.

But whether you decide to keep saturated fat in your diet or not, you will benefit by swapping it out (at least occasionally) for the fats identified as "good" fats.

Unsaturated fats, aka "good fats," can be either monounsaturated or polyunsaturated. Both mono- and polyunsaturated fats have been found to promote heart health when consumed in moderation.

Specifically, mono- and polyunsaturated have been shown to raise "good" cholesterol in the body, called high-density lipoprotein (HDL). Higher levels of HDL are associated with a lower risk of heart disease.

Another benefit of polyunsaturated fats is that they contain omega-3 fatty acids. Omega-3s are found in fatty fish (like tuna, trout, and salmon) and in some seeds, like flaxseed. You can also take omega-3 fatty acids in supplement form.

TECHNICAL STUFF

Omega-3 fatty acids have been associated with a wide range of health benefits, including a lower risk of certain cancers, heart disease, Alzheimer's disease, dementia, and age-related macular degeneration (AMD).

Consider adding some mono- and polyunsaturated foods to your meals.

Foods with monounsaturated fats include:

>> Avocado

>> Canola oil

>> Nuts

>> Olive oil

>> Peanut oil and butter

>> Safflower oil (high oleic)

>> Sesame oil

>> Sunflower oil

Foods with polyunsaturated fats include:

- » Corn oil
- » Fish, such as salmon, mackerel, herring, albacore tuna, and trout
- » Flaxseeds or flax oil
- » Safflower oil
- » Soybean oil
- » Sunflower seeds
- » Walnuts

The bottom line is that fat plays a key role in good health. It is rich in calories, so if weight loss or weight maintenance is your goal, then you should consume it in moderation. Filling your grocery cart with healthy fat foods like nuts, seeds, avocado, plant-based oils, and fatty fish can help you to stay full and satisfied while potentially boosting your health.

Micronutrients Are Important, Too: Vitamins and Minerals

If macros are the large building blocks of nutrition, then micronutrients — vitamins and minerals — are the tiny building blocks. Your body needs vitamins and minerals in very small amounts, but they are no less important than macronutrients.

REMEMBER

Except for vitamin D, your body cannot produce most vitamins and minerals, so they must be consumed in the diet. Micronutrients are vital to growth development, disease prevention, and overall wellness.

Going on the macro diet may help you to increase your intake of these important nutrients.

The macro diet encourages you to plan meals and eat a variety of foods, especially nutrient-rich grains, fruits, vegetables, and healthy oils. All of these foods are high in both macro and micronutrients. Processed foods generally contain fewer vitamins and minerals.

Some people take a multivitamin to ensure they get the nutrients they need. But health experts advise that you get vitamins and minerals from food rather than supplements. Food comes bundled with other nutrients, like fiber, protein, or omega-3 fatty acids. Also, multivitamins are not regulated the way you think they might be.

According to the National Institutes of Health (NIH), no standard or regulatory definition for multivitamins or multi-vitamin and mineral supplements (such as what nutrients they must contain or in what amounts) exists, so you can't always rely on a particular formula or product to give you the nutrition you need.

Government health organizations, like the NIH, provide recommendations about how much of each micronutrient you should consume each day. These recommendations vary based on your gender and age. Other variables may come into play as well.

You can use NIH recommendations as your starting point for establishing what vitamins and minerals you need. If you want personalized advice, speak to your healthcare provider or get a referral to a registered dietitian (RD).

Important vitamins and common sources

If you want to track your intake of certain vitamins or minerals, you can probably use the same tracking app that you are using to track your macros. For example, apps (and websites) like MyFitnessPal allow you to choose a few nutrients to track outside of your macros. Chapter 7 provides a rundown of different tracking methods.

If you are using a pen and paper method, you can use the Nutrition Facts label to find out if a food contains a significant amount of a particular vitamin or mineral. Keep in mind, however, that food manufacturers are not required to list vitamins or minerals on the label.

Daily values (DV) are listed for several vitamins and minerals in Table 2-1. Daily Values are the recommended amounts of nutrients to consume or not to exceed each day. Table 2-1 is not a comprehensive list of every vitamin but a list of the vitamins the NIH identifies as essential for good health. Keep in mind that nutrient intake for infants, children, and teens is often different than it is for adults.

Important minerals and common sources

In addition to vitamins, certain minerals are needed for good health. The two different types of minerals are macrominerals and trace minerals.

>> **Macrominerals** are needed in larger amounts. These minerals include calcium, phosphorus, magnesium, sodium, potassium, chloride, and sulfur.

>> **Trace minerals** are needed in smaller amounts. They include iron, manganese, copper, iodine, zinc, cobalt, fluoride, and selenium.

TABLE 2-1 **Daily Values of Select Nutrients**

Vitamin	Recommended Intake	Food Sources
Vitamin A	900 micrograms (mcg)	Colorful fruits and veggies, liver, whole milk, and some cereals
B vitamins (thiamine, riboflavin, niacin, pantothenic acid, biotin, vitamin B-6, vitamin B-12 and folate)	Varies based on specific nutrient	Fish, poultry, meat, eggs, dairy products, leafy green vegetables, beans, and peas
Vitamin C	90 milligrams (mg)	Citrus fruit, red and green peppers, tomatoes, broccoli, and green leafy veggies
Vitamin D	20mcg	Sun exposure, egg yolks, saltwater fish, and liver
Vitamin E	15mg	Nuts and seeds, leafy greens, vegetable oils
Vitamin K	120mcg	Green vegetables and dark berries

The FDA provides recommended intakes for each mineral. They vary based on your gender, age, and other factors such as stage of life.

For instance, post-menopausal women may need more calcium than younger adult men and women. Your sodium intake may need to be limited if you have or are at risk for hypertension. Again, your healthcare provider or registered dietitian is the best source for learning more about your personalized needs.

TIP

You'll get minerals in many of the same healthy foods that provide vitamins, including nuts, beans, lentils, dark leafy greens, fish, seeds, shellfish, and whole grains.

Hydration and the Macro Diet

The last nutrient you should concern yourself with is water. Water accounts for about 60 percent of your total body weight. Staying hydrated contributes to your health in so many ways.

Water is essential for metabolism, the transport of nutrients across membranes, cell health, temperature regulation, and proper circulatory function. And staying hydrated helps you to feel strong and energized!

Not getting enough fluids, on the other hand, can lead to dehydration. Severe dehydration can cause symptoms such as confusion, fainting, rapid heartbeat, and rapid breathing. But even mild dehydration can cause symptoms.

If you're even mildly dehydrated, you may feel sluggish, thirsty, headachy, and your skin and mouth may feel dry. You may also feel hungry when you are dehydrated.

So how do you know if you're getting enough fluids to stay hydrated? Recommendations and guidelines vary, so it is important to familiarize yourself with them. Your water needs may vary from day to day.

Intake guidelines for water

Most people don't think about their water intake. Most of us drink when thirsty and often drink water with meals to make eating easier. But tracking your water intake isn't a bad idea, especially if you struggle with hunger or fatigue.

TIP

Several fitness and nutrition apps help you to track your water intake. You may want to track yours for a week or so to see how it compares to recommended levels. You may find that increasing your fluid intake helps you to avoid fatigue or food cravings.

In terms of the amount of water to drink, you might think of the age-old recommendation: eight glasses per day. That's not a bad place to start, but health organizations like the National Academy of Medicine suggest drinking more.

REMEMBER

Adequate fluid intake is considered to be 13 cups (104 ounces) per day for men and 9 cups (72 ounces) for women, according to the National Academy of Medicine.

Children and teens need a little bit less than adults, and people who are pregnant or breastfeeding will need more. If you are ill (fever or vomiting), you will need more fluids to maintain proper hydration.

TIP

You can also use the color of your urine to make sure you're getting enough to drink. When your urine is very light yellow, you are probably getting enough fluids. But when it starts to turn dark, you may be dehydrated. However, some supplements also darken your urine, so this is not always the most accurate method.

Also, remember that when you exercise, you'll need to increase your fluid intake. Sweating rids your body of water, and those fluids must be replaced. As a general rule, you should plan to consume 0.4 to 0.8 liters (13.5 to 27 ounces) per hour when you are doing vigorous exercise for an hour or more.

You can also estimate your fluid needs by weighing yourself before and after exercise (ensure you have not eaten before the weigh-in). You'll notice that your weight has decreased from fluid loss. At your next exercise session, use that number as a guide for how much fluid to consume.

Tips for staying hydrated

While most of us think of hydrating with water, you can get your fluid levels up to recommended levels in many other ways. Use these tips to stay hydrated and healthy throughout the day.

- » **Choose water-filled fruits and veggies.** Melon, berries, pineapple, peaches, leafy greens, broccoli, bell peppers, and celery can help you stay hydrated.

- » **Drink a glass of water in the morning** before you have your coffee. Have a glass of water before bed, and consider keeping a water bottle on your nightstand to hydrate during the night.

- » **Grab a little extra water if you're eating salty foods.** Drinking water helps to neutralize the sodium, and the thirst you feel when you eat salty food is a good reminder to drink up!

- » **Keep a water bottle handy** in your car, at the office, on your desk at work, and on the coffee table when you're watching television or reading in the evening. The bottle helps to serve as a reminder to drink.

- » **Pre-fill your water for the following day** and keep those bottles in the fridge next to your macro-prepped meals. Commit to emptying the entire amount throughout the day.

- » **Use flavors to your advantage** if you don't like the taste of water. Add cucumber, melon balls, berries, citrus fruit, or basil to flavor water. You can also buy flavor tablets.

Lastly, be mindful of your body's cues throughout the day. Dehydration can sometimes feel like hunger or sleepiness. If you find yourself wanting a snack (especially if it is shortly after eating), have a glass of water first and see if that curbs the craving. Similarly, when you feel that late-afternoon energy slump hit, grab your water bottle and slug a few gulps. Better yet, if you know the slump is coming, hydrate in the hours before it hits. You may find that you gain greater energy from simply drinking more fluids.

» **Seeing how the macro diet contributes to overall health and longevity**

» **Understanding how the nutritional strategy supports fitness, athletic, and body composition goals**

» **Making weight loss manageable and healthy with the macro diet**

» **Honing skills for a lifetime of wellness**

Chapter **3**

Enjoying the Benefits of a Macro Diet

C hanging your diet to balance your macronutrient intake can offer a wide range of benefits. The benefits that you enjoy may depend on how you approach the diet. While one person might see quick changes in a short period of time, others may see a steady stream of beneficial effects that show up (and remain consistent) over the long term.

In this chapter, I explain the various benefits of the macro diet. I show you how understanding the techniques outlined in this book can impact your overall wellness and even have an impact on your long-term nutritional health, regardless of whether or not you continue to track your macros consistently.

Knowing the many benefits of the macro diet sets you up for a positive experience on your journey to a healthier lifestyle by helping you acknowledge your progress, stick to your plan, or make adjustments that serve your personalized needs.

Increasing Nutritional Awareness

Knowledge is power! On the macro diet, you learn more about nutrition in general, but you also gain a better understanding of your body's personalized needs, which can empower you to make food choices that benefit your health.

Macronutrients play an important role in your overall health. Experiencing the macro diet shows you which foods contain each macro and about how to make healthy choices when shopping for different types of foods. In addition, I provide you with the latest guidelines from various health organizations about how much of each macro to consume each day.

You can put all of this information to use in developing your own macro diet plan to reach your personalized goals. And that's when you can take your nutritional knowledge to the next level.

TIP

As you try out your new macro diet, you can see how your body adapts to different macro ratios. Then, you can make adjustments according to how you feel.

For example, maybe your original macro diet plan includes a carbohydrate-rich morning meal because you enjoy breakfast foods that are higher in carbs, like pancakes or a bagel. But after following the diet for a couple of weeks, a pattern emerges that you'd like to fix — you experience an energy slump after a few hours of eating.

The macro diet shows you that choosing foods with protein and fiber can give your breakfast staying power. So, adding an egg to your breakfast and choosing a whole-grain bagel instead of one made with white flour is the way to go.

In this scenario, your new breakfast plan still honors your food preferences, but you've adjusted the macro balance of the meal by adding different foods. *Voilà!* You've solved your energy slump issue.

REMEMBER

On the macro diet, you become an expert in your own nutritional needs. You develop an arsenal of information that you can use to make healthy food and meal decisions that serve your needs.

Your improved nutritional awareness may also help you to steer clear of the many unhealthy diet trends and fads that infiltrate magazines, TV, and social media. There is certainly no shortage of them; you've probably seen the mushroom diet, the grapefruit diet, the mono diet, and on and on and on.

But when you understand the importance of balanced nutrition, it becomes easier to avoid fad diets that suggest limiting or entirely eliminating certain macronutrients. You can feel confident in knowing that while diet trends may come and go, a balanced diet with adequate protein, carbohydrates, and fat has stood the test of time.

Enhancing Overall Well-Being

Putting your nutritional focus on balanced macronutrients can support both your physical and emotional well-being. While countless supplements and other products sold in health and vitamin stores claim to elevate your health, a foundational approach to your diet may have a more lasting and meaningful impact.

TECHNICAL STUFF

A 2020 report published in the journal *Nutrients* highlights how macronutrients contribute to our diet, explaining that proportional macronutrient intake is inextricably linked to health and longevity. The report explains that there is no single macro balance that is known to be the "right" combination and emphasizes that different proportions have been used to address various health issues around the world.

Adapting your macros to align with the healthy eating pattern identified by the Dietary Guidelines for Americans (DGA — see Chapter 6 for more details) can also lower your risk for certain diseases. According to the U.S. Centers for Disease Control and Prevention, people with healthy eating patterns are at lower risk for serious health problems such as heart disease, type 2 diabetes, and obesity.

And your mental well-being might also get a boost from following the macro diet. Knowing how to adjust the way your body feels throughout the day or performs at the gym is likely to give you a sense of empowerment and improved confidence. Not only that, but you may be able to develop a healthier relationship with food.

REMEMBER

On the macro diet, no foods are "good," and no foods are "bad." All foods contribute to your health and happiness in one way or another. There is no such thing as "cheating" on this diet and no reason to feel guilt or shame for choosing one food over another.

For many people, this freedom from food judgment may provide a welcome relief. It is not unusual for diet programs, especially weight-loss diets, to provide a list of non-compliant foods. If a food that you enjoy is on that list, you may feel deprived or, worse yet, bad about yourself if you eat it. But on the macro diet, your only goal is to find balance.

Improving Fitness and Sports Performance

The macro diet tends to be very popular among athletes and fitness enthusiasts who use it to reach specific performance goals. A balanced macronutrient diet can help you train better and get more out of your workouts.

TIP

Countless studies have demonstrated how getting adequate amounts of protein, fat, and carbohydrates contributes to athletic training and competition. You can use the macro diet to make sure your dietary intake meets guidelines set by sports nutrition experts to maximize results.

Maximizing muscle gain with protein

If you are a strength-trained athlete, getting enough protein is absolutely essential if you want to make the most of your time in the weight room. Without important amino acids from protein-rich foods, your body won't have the building blocks it needs to repair and build muscle tissue.

Sports nutrition experts provide very specific guidelines for the amount of protein to consume to maximize muscle gains (provided for you in Chapter 6). On the macro diet, you learn how to plan meals and track the grams of protein you consume each day to ensure you meet these recommendations.

Can you just increase your protein intake without the macro diet to get more protein for muscle-building? Well, yes. But without a tracking system in place, it may not be successful. Researchers have consistently found that most people are not very good at remembering what they eat.

I DIDN'T EAT THAT!

Several studies have demonstrated that people have a tendency to underreport their caloric intake. That is, they think they are eating less than they actually eat. But for some macros, like protein, there are interesting gender differences.

One study suggested that when it comes to macros, people might overreport their intake. The study involved just under 250 men and women. Study authors found that women were fairly accurate in estimating the amount of protein that they consumed, but men were not. In fact, men overreported their protein intake by 12 percent to 19 percent.

That level of inaccuracy can make a big difference if you are a guy who is working hard on a weight-training program. Every gram of protein matters to your muscles!

The planning and tracking systems built into the macro diet help you to be more precise about your nutrient intake so that your hard work in the gym is well supported by your diet.

Eating for endurance

It is not just weightlifters who can reap nutritional rewards on the macro diet. Those who participate in aerobic and endurance activities also gain advantages when they measure and track their intake of macros. Whether you are a serious runner, an aerobic dance enthusiast, or a stair-climbing fanatic, getting adequate carbs can ensure that you have the energy you need to crush your workout.

Organizations like the American College of Sports Medicine (ACSM) provide nutritional recommendations for athletes and fitness enthusiasts. They remind us that most of our energy (at least 50 percent of total calories) should come from nutrient-dense "real food" carbohydrates to fuel both day-to-day activities and exercise.

When you adopt the macro diet, you can plan ahead to add carb-rich foods like whole grains, vegetables, fruits, nuts, and seeds to each meal to spread out your carbohydrate intake throughout the day. By tracking your intake, you'll have the confidence of knowing you're giving your body the fuel it needs.

The result is that you'll have steady energy for simple tasks like gardening, walking through the parking lot, and carrying groceries into the house, but you'll also have plenty of gusto left to power through your gym session.

Amplifying fitness benefits with fat

There are clear benefits to getting enough fat in your diet, whether you are a strength-trained athlete, an endurance athlete, or simply a workout junkie. Getting enough healthy fat in amounts that align with DGA guidelines can provide a few benefits.

Several studies, including a 2022 systematic review published in the journal *Nutrients*, identify how getting high-quality fatty acids (such as omega-3 fatty acids) can provide advantages, such as:

>> Maintaining optimal hormone levels (especially testosterone)

>> Reducing muscle soreness and inflammation after workouts or competition

>> Reducing muscle atrophy during periods of injury (in combination with protein and carbohydrates)

But researchers also point out, however, that getting too much fat can be detrimental.

On the macro diet, you monitor how much fat you consume each day. Planning your meals in advance and meal prep strategies can also help you to make more careful choices about the type of fat you consume so that you can take advantage of the nutritional benefits of consuming high-quality fats.

When you first start out on the macro diet, you may not want to track and monitor your intake of *each* macronutrient (protein, fat, and carbs). But that is the great thing about this diet plan. You can target one macro to start with and build from there.

For example, if you have started a weight-training program, you might start by monitoring your protein intake to maximize its muscle-building properties. Then, as you get comfortable with skills such as tracking macros, planning meals, and food prep, you can begin to target and track other nutrients as you feel comfortable. Eventually, you'll have a well-rounded food plan that you can feel good about and that helps your body perform at its best.

Promoting Better Body Composition

Body composition refers to the ratio of fat mass to lean tissue (such as bone and muscle) on your body. Body composition is often measured in terms of body fat percentage.

In many ways, body composition is a better measurement of health and fitness than body weight. When you simply weigh yourself, the number on the scale can't tell you how much of your body is strong muscle and bone, but body fat percentage can.

Different organizations, like the American Council on Exercise (ACE) and the National Association of Sports Medicine (NASM), provide norms and body fat ranges to help you understand where your body fat range might fall. Experts in other countries use similar numbers. For example, HealthLink BC (based in British Columbia) suggests that 10 to 22 percent body fat is considered healthy in an adult man, and 20 to 32 percent body fat is considered healthy in an adult woman.

The numbers listed in Table 3-1 are not necessarily recommendations but simply typical ranges for different types of people.

TABLE 3-1

Body Fat Percentage Categories

Description	Women	Men
Essential body fat	10% to 13%	2% to 5%
Body fat for athletes	14% to 20%	6% to 13%
Fitness-level body fat	21% to 24%	14% to 17%
Acceptable body fat	25% to 31%	18% to 24%
Body fat level considered obese	More than 32%	More than 25%

A number of different factors can impact your body fat percentage, such as age, fitness level, and lifestyle. And it is important to note that less body fat is not necessarily better.

REMEMBER

You need fat on your body for insulation, to protect vital organs, and to provide energy. Your body won't perform well athletically if you don't have adequate fat. But having too much body fat has also been associated with certain health conditions such as high blood pressure, heart disease, and diabetes.

For these reasons, some people prefer to change their body fat percentage rather than just targeting their weight.

Simply restricting calories to lose weight may help you lose body fat, but it can also lead to the loss of strong muscle tissue. However, using a targeted macro diet can help you preserve valuable muscle mass while diminishing body fat to your desired range.

Getting enough protein can help you build muscle mass when combined with a weight-training program. But getting adequate protein is also important for your muscles when you are trying to reduce your body fat.

Numerous studies have shown that adequate protein intake can help preserve muscle mass during weight loss. And having more muscle mass can help you to maintain a better metabolic rate for general health or fat loss.

For instance, a 2021 review published in the journal *Nutrients* explains that while cutting calories along with exercise is the most common method used for weight loss, this combined approach can negatively impact body composition, specifically muscle mass.

The review's authors explain that losing muscle can also impact metabolic health and the quality and quantity of life, especially in post-menopausal women, older adults, athletes, and those with metabolic disease. To combat this type of muscle loss, they suggest consuming protein at an intake level greater than the current guideline of 0.8 grams per kilogram of body weight per day.

I explain the current guidelines for protein intake in Chapter 6, so you can decide how much to consume for your lifestyle and your goals. But the best way to know that you're getting enough protein is to plan and track your intake with the macro diet.

REMEMBER

When you plan and track meals on the macro diet, you can be sure to add healthy protein-rich foods, like eggs, lean meat, legumes, and protein-rich veggies (like spinach) to your meals. This approach to nutrition helps you to optimize nutrient intake so you can maintain optimum body composition to perform well in athletics and age with vigor.

Reaching and Maintaining a Healthy Weight

Weight loss is one of the most common reasons that people become interested in the macro diet. This diet (or any diet for that matter) is not a magic bullet for weight loss. But the macro diet can definitely help you reach a healthy target weight if that is your goal. In fact, I would argue that it can be the healthiest and most accurate method for reaching your weight-loss goals.

TECHNICAL STUFF

According to media reports, about 45 million Americans go on a diet every year. Many of those dieters choose to go on some sort of commercial diet or restrictive program where they are required to cut out or significantly reduce their intake of certain types of foods or even entire food groups. Unfortunately, those programs are not highly successful. About 65 percent of dieters return to their pre-diet weight within three years.

The macro diet is not a restrictive plan, but it can still promote healthy and sustainable weight loss by focusing on balanced nutrition. When you consume adequate amounts of protein, fat, and carbohydrates, you don't get the hunger, fatigue, and feelings of deprivation that often accompany traditional weight-loss programs.

REMEMBER

What makes the macro diet different from traditional weight-loss diets is that your focus will be on getting *enough* of each food group rather than cutting back or cutting out certain foods. The emphasis each day will be on reaching your macro targets, so your tank is always full of good nutrition.

By putting the emphasis on macros, you set yourself up for success. Each macronutrient helps support your weight loss progress in a different way. In this section, I show you how getting enough of each macronutrient matters for weight loss and why tracking your intake is the best way to ensure you meet balanced and healthy targets.

Boosting your metabolism with protein

Getting enough protein has been shown in numerous studies to promote weight loss and long-term weight maintenance.

For instance, a 2020 research review published in the *Journal of Obesity and Metabolic Syndrome* reports significant clinical evidence demonstrates that a high-protein diet provides weight-loss effects and can prevent weight regain after weight loss. The review authors even called out one study in which participants followed a macro-style diet.

In the study, participants could eat whatever they wanted at several different restaurants, but they had to adhere to specific macronutrient goals (just like the macro diet). Some participants had to consume a higher protein diet (25 percent of calories from protein), while others had to reach higher carb or higher fat targets.

At the end of six months, those who consumed the higher protein diet lost more weight than those who followed the higher carb or higher fat plan. And what's even more interesting is that the study authors noted a lower dropout rate with this type of macro tracking program than in typical diets.

So how does getting enough protein to promote weight loss? Researchers suggest that consuming adequate protein can help you to maintain or even increase your total daily energy expenditure (TDEE), which is the total number of calories you burn each day. (Chapter 6 gives you the details on TDEE.)

REMEMBER

Eating protein helps you to burn more calories from diet-induced energy expenditure, also called the thermic effect of food. This is the amount of energy (calories) needed to digest and metabolize food. It takes more energy to process protein than it does to process fat or carbohydrate.

The scientists also noted that consuming more protein can improve your metabolic rate when your body is at rest or sleeping. (*Metabolic rate* is the rate at which your body burns calories.) And, finally, the study authors pointed to the fact that protein improves *satiety* or the feeling of fullness.

With all of these benefits to offer, making sure you consume adequate protein is a smart priority if your goal is to lose weight. Tracking your macros is the smartest way to make sure you reach your targets to gain these benefits.

Crushing fatigue with adequate carbs

Getting enough protein shouldn't mean cutting out carbs and fat, which is often recommended on traditional diets. On the macro diet it's all about balance!

Carbohydrates are your body's preferred energy source. While you can use fat or protein for energy, your body feels better when you consume the right amount of carbs. (For a more detailed explanation, see Chapter 2.)

So, what about all of those low-carb diets you see mentioned in magazines and on social media? Low-carb diets have gained attention in recent years because they can result in short-term weight loss, often due to water loss. But low-carb diets are often unsustainable in the long run, because they can lead to uncomfortable symptoms, like fatigue.

In scientific studies, low carbohydrate diets have been associated with symptoms including nausea, fatigue, water and electrolyte losses, and limits on exercise capacity.

Alternatively, diets that are too high in carbs can result in large swings in your body's insulin levels, which may cause increased hunger and calorie consumption, according to the National Institutes of Health.

On the macro diet, you set goals for your carb intake based on the latest nutritional guidelines. Then, you track your intake each day to make sure you reach your carbohydrate sweet spot: not too low and not too high. Doing so will help you to enjoy steady energy levels throughout the day without increased hunger or cravings.

Feeling full and satisfied with fat

Not surprisingly, tracking your fat intake can help you to slim down. Fat provides nine calories per gram while carbs and protein each provide only four calories per gram.

Since fat is more calorie-dense, it is important to make sure you aren't overconsuming it if your goal is weight loss. But your body *needs* fat, so it's also important that you get enough.

Fat is important for healthy cells, but more importantly, fat makes food taste good and helps us to enjoy eating. Fat helps us to feel full and happy after eating. If you want your weight-loss program to be sustainable, getting the right amount of fat is key.

Of course, the macro diet isn't the only way to ensure that you get fat, carbs, and protein in your diet. You can pay for a commercial meal service in which all of the food is premeasured and provided for you (often for a hefty price). But macro tracking puts you in control. And dietary tracking has been shown in scientific studies to enhance weight-loss efforts.

TECHNICAL STUFF

A 2017 study published in the *Journal of Diabetes Research* suggests that frequent dietary tracking is an important component of long-term weight loss success. Specifically, researchers found that tracking at least five days per week led to more significant and sustained weight loss over time as compared to tracking fewer days or tracking inconsistently.

On the macro diet, you take control of your daily nutrition so that you feel empowered to make food choices that support your goal, whether it is weight loss, weight gain, or improved health. The tracking process can help you to feel empowered while also giving you the confidence of knowing you are providing your body with the nutrients it needs to be strong and healthy.

Supporting a Lifelong Strategy for Wellness

Because you design the macro diet to work according to your own lifestyle, it is a much more sustainable program than many other diets out there. You can use this program throughout a lifetime of change in whatever way supports your current needs.

Several different factors make the diet sustainable, including the fact that there is no fixed timeline, it's budget-friendly, it isn't socially restrictive, it can be used intermittently, and it supports a wide variety of goals.

Flexible timeline

One of the great things about the macro diet is that it doesn't require a major immediate shift in your dietary habits. You can completely overhaul your diet right away if you want to, but you certainly don't have to.

On many diets — especially weight-loss diets — change is immediate and substantial because there is a timeline advertised for losing weight. That works for some people. They like the "clean slate" that a fresh start affords them. And the idea of reaching a goal on a specific date can be appealing. But sometimes, that kind of change can feel harsh and is not sustainable.

Since the macro diet is set up to be a long-term approach to nutrition, there is no need to hurry up and make major alterations to the way you eat. In fact, gradual change might work better.

Gradual change can help you to adapt to new foods, new tastes, or new portion sizes with greater ease. And gradual adjustments can make the benefits easier to track.

For example, after you figure out your macro numbers, you might choose to target one macronutrient at a time. Let's say that you decide that you want to increase your carb intake so that it is in line with recommended guidelines. You decide that you want to do so by increasing your consumption of whole grains.

Shopping for whole grains might be new for you and might require a little bit of extra time at the grocery store. You'll need to read package labels more carefully and scan the Nutrition Facts label. It may be less stressful for you to tackle this step if you aren't also tasked with shopping for new protein foods and different types of healthy fats.

In addition, as you incorporate those whole grains into your diet, you will notice changes and know that they are the result of the carb shift.

You might notice steadier energy levels after eating. You might notice better bowel habits (fiber-rich foods can help to normalize bowel movements). You may experience fewer sugar cravings throughout the day.

By changing one factor at a time, it is easier to identify which dietary change is benefiting you (or not).

On the macro diet, you choose the timeline and approach that works best for you. If you have a short-term goal that you want to reach, you can completely rebuild your diet on day one. But if you prefer a more moderate pace for lifelong sustainability, that works as well.

Budget-friendly

Another benefit that contributes to the sustainability of the macro diet is the fact that it can be budget-friendly. You don't need to pay for a commercial diet plan or food subscription. There is also no need to buy expensive or trendy foods. Since all foods are compliant on this diet, you can shop within your means.

TIP

In fact, many people buy in bulk when they prep meals in advance for the macro diet. This can help you save substantially, especially over the long term.

The budget-friendly nature of the macro diet may be especially important if you experience major changes in your life like a job loss, a new baby, going back to school, or a move to a new state.

Even if you aren't experiencing financial hardship, saving money is always appealing. The macro diet can not only improve your physical health, but it can contribute to your financial health as well.

Easy in social situations

If you're on the macro diet, there is no need to make special accommodations in social situations. On some diets where certain foods are off limits, going out to dinner, going to a party, or going on a date might be challenging if food is involved. There may not be food available that fits within your meal plan. In addition, it can be awkward to explain to others why you are not eating certain foods.

On the macro diet, you eat what you want. All foods contain at least one and usually several macros. So, you can enjoy food in any social situation without the worry of explaining your diet to others or offending those who have cooked for you.

So, what happens if the food served doesn't align exactly with your macro targets? Or what if you don't know the exact nutritional make-up of the food that is served? You can either make adjustments at your next meal to bring your nutrient totals in line, or you can simply skip counting for that day or that meal. Since the macro diet is a meal plan for life, a single meal here or a day off there isn't going to do any damage.

TIP

You can *and should* continue to enjoy all of the food-related social situations that you did before starting the program. Continuing to enjoy your life and enjoying the company of others around food is part of what makes this plan sustainable.

Intermittent use

One of my favorite features of the macro diet is that you can use the diet for a period of time, then dial it back a bit, and then go back on it again.

You will probably set up your initial plan to reach a specific goal. During that time, you track your nutrients and plan meals according to specific targets. But once you reach your goal, you can either set a new goal and continue tracking, or you can back off from tracking and planning and then track occasionally moving forward just to make sure that you aren't veering too far from your initial targets.

For instance, perhaps you are training to run a marathon. You set up a macro diet that prioritizes carbohydrate intake so that you've got plenty of energy for those long training runs and for race day. You track your macros meticulously to ensure the proper balance of nutrition.

When race day is over, you may not want to spend as much time or energy watching your macros. And your carb intake still matters, but it is not as essential as it was during training. So, you might skip the tracking component of the macro diet and just plan meals around a general balance of macros instead. Or, you might use one of the alternate macro strategies that I offer in Chapter 12.

Every once in a while, you can track your nutrient intake for a week or so just to be sure that you are getting macronutrients in ranges that are healthy. For example, perhaps you notice a change in your health, such as lower energy levels or a change in your weight. You can track your macros for a week or two to see how it compares to your previous nutrient intake. If you see that there are significant discrepancies, you might go back to meal planning and tracking for a while to get yourself back on track.

TIP

This kind of flexibility can make sticking to your program a little easier when you are in the more stringent phases of your plan. If you know that you don't have to count and track every food you eat for life, then it can be easier to stay on track for the short term.

There is no specific goal or endpoint

There is nothing wrong with diets that have a specific target in mind. For instance, the DASH diet (Dietary Approaches to Stop Hypertension) is often prescribed for people who want to bring their blood pressure down or reduce their risk for heart disease. These diets have been shown to be highly successful in meeting specific goals.

But there is also value in having a nutritional plan that can be set up to meet any goal. It means that as your priorities and circumstances change throughout life, your diet can change with you.

On the macro diet, you decide what healthy looks like for you. You set the bar for success and decide when you have reached your goal.

You also get to decide how to move forward. Perhaps you decide to take on new nutritional adventures. Maybe you want to try a plant-based diet or see what it is like to go gluten-free or eat paleo foods. Or perhaps your healthcare provider has suggested a diet to address medical issues.

The macro diet is flexible enough to work well with almost any nutritional strategy. It is highly adaptable. The skills you develop in this program are skills that help you to follow any other diet plan for any health or fitness goal.

As you work through this book, try to keep these various benefits in mind. You may even find that journaling and noting the benefits you experience is helpful. Knowing how far you have come and keeping track of your successes is a great way to support yourself on your nutritional journey.

Chapter **4**

Deciding if the Macro Diet Is Right for You

The macro diet is an eating plan (and a lifestyle!) that works for people with different goals and throughout different stages of life. But no diet works for everyone. The macro diet, just like every other diet, may not be the right fit for some people. So, it is important to examine both the advantages and potential concerns about this or any new meal plan.

REMEMBER

Your needs are unique. What works for one person may not always work for another. It is never a good idea to start a diet just because someone you know or a celebrity or social media influencer says that they are on that diet. Their circumstances and their goals may be substantially different from yours.

When considering any diet plan, you can also talk to your healthcare provider to see how it might affect any health conditions you have. In some cases, you may be able to adjust the diet to meet your personalized needs.

For instance, if you are at risk for type 2 diabetes and you adopt the macro diet, you'll want to choose carbs carefully and spread out your intake to keep your blood sugar levels stable throughout the day.

TIP

If your healthcare provider is not well versed in this eating plan or if their background in nutrition is limited, ask for a referral to a registered dietitian (RD) or a registered dietitian nutritionist (RDN). An RD or RDN can help you set up your plan and give you personalized guidance about how this plan will affect your current health status.

In this chapter, I go into detail about the best candidates for the macro diet, such as those who love food and enjoy the benefits of good nutrition. I also provide information about those who should be cautious when choosing this plan. I walk you through the pros and cons and provide tips so that you can make the best decision for you about the macro diet.

The Best Candidates for a Macro Diet

Because the macro diet is a flexible diet, the range of people who can be successful on this plan is wide. That said, some people are especially well-suited for this plan.

People who prioritize good nutrition

If eating a delicious and healthy meal makes you feel good, then you're likely to do well on this plan. And if you appreciate the benefits of common-sense nutrition, then the macro diet is definitely for you.

The macro diet can also be the perfect partner to other types of diet plans, such as those that focus on food type (such as a plant-based diet, Mediterranean diet, or the paleo diet — see Chapter 1 for more on these diets). The macro diet dovetails well with these food plans to ensure you get the right ratio of macronutrients.

TIP

If you already invest time and energy into a particular eating style, then you're a great candidate for the macro diet. You've already prioritized good nutrition and may have many of the skills that make the macro diet work. Counting your macros will just ensure that you're getting the best ratio of protein, fat, and carbs.

For instance, maybe you've decided to go vegan and consume only plant-based foods. Just choosing vegan foods doesn't necessarily guarantee that you will get protein, fat, and carbs in the recommended amounts. In fact, some vegans and vegetarians struggle to get enough protein.

But choosing to go vegan requires that you put extra time and careful consideration into your food choices. These skills make the macro diet easier to follow. And when you add macro tracking to your existing vegan plan, you'll ensure that you get all of the protein, fat, and carbs you need to stay healthy.

People who enjoy reaching goals

If you are a goal-oriented person, you will do well on the macro diet because the entire program is based on your personalized aspirations and interests.

Goal-oriented people gain confidence by identifying clear objectives, monitoring their progress, and finally crossing the finish line. They harness the power of accomplishment to fuel new adventures and tackle new challenges.

On the macro diet, every day is a new opportunity to set and reach nutritional goals. Every day, you track your progress and make adjustments to reach protein, fat, and carb targets. At the end of the day, you can celebrate your efforts, knowing that you helped your body stay strong and healthy.

TIP

If goal setting is new to you, you're also a good candidate for this program. In Chapter 5, I go over everything you need to know to set a SMART goal, the type of goal that has been shown in clinical and business settings to be effective — even for newbies. You'll be able to set smaller short-term goals to build your confidence and then raise the bar as you become goal-savvy.

People who like to be organized

If you like the extra time (and mental sanity) that good organization can provide, then you'll feel right at home on the macro diet. Like any good organizational plan, it takes a bit more work upfront but allows you to relax and go into autopilot after the program is set up.

Macro diet meal prep is the ultimate food organization system. It reduces the hard work (and stress) of decision-making at mealtime and can reduce your overall workload in the kitchen. In Chapter 8, I show you how to set up your kitchen, shop for macro foods, and prep meals like a pro.

And if you are an organized person who likes data, you'll enjoy tracking your numbers on the macro diet even more. If you like charts and measurements, then this meal plan will work especially well for you. The macro diet is all about making sure you reach your targets every day.

But don't worry, you don't have to be a numbers whiz to make this program work. There are many different ways to track your macros on this diet, so even if you don't consider yourself to be a numbers person, you'll still be able to find an organized tracking system that works for you.

TIP

You can use an app, make a colorful chart to hang in your kitchen, or carry a journal to record your food data. In Chapter 11, I even offer a few tracking-free ways to take advantage of this program if you don't want to do any math.

People who like food

Last but (definitely) not least, this program is great for people who like food. Food makes us happy! If you like cooking food, preparing food, thinking about food, or, most importantly, eating food, you'll feel satisfied on the macro diet.

There are many different ways to get the nutrients your body needs to perform in life and sport. In fact, the supplement industry makes billions of dollars every year selling pills, potions, and powders that promise to deliver benefits to make you stronger, smarter, faster, and healthier. However, nutrition experts continue to recommend that you get your nutrition primarily from food rather than supplements.

Supplements can't provide your body with optimized nutrition the way that whole food can. And supplements usually don't taste good! On the macro diet, you get to enjoy tasty meals while ensuring that you get the nutrition that you need.

REMEMBER

That being said, if you choose to use a supplement (such as a protein powder or a multivitamin), you know that you are *building* on a solid foundation of good nutrition rather than relying on that supplement to make up for less-than-perfect diet choices.

Whether your goal is athletic performance, weight loss, or improved health, why not enjoy meals that are both delicious and nutritious with the satisfaction of knowing you are following evidence-based guidance to support your goals? The macro diet is the perfect approach for food lovers.

Who Should Exercise Caution When Considering a Macro Diet

Although the macro diet works well for most people, it is not the best plan for certain types of people, such as those looking for a quick fix, those with a strained relationship with food, or those at risk for developing an eating disorder.

Anyone looking for a quick fix

The macro diet tends to be most appealing to people who are tired of restrictive eating plans or fad diets that only allow them to eat certain foods. If you are looking for a quick fix, a "cleanse," or a short-term detox program, then the macro diet will disappoint you.

For instance, if you are looking for a super-fast way to slim down, you're not likely to find this program very successful. But guess what? No quick-fix weight loss program works. We know from study after study that even if the weight comes off in the short term, it comes back in the long run (and usually brings some extra pounds with it).

If weight loss is your goal, the macro diet will work well when you are looking for steady, consistent progress. But if you're looking for a quickie slim down, then the macro diet is probably not for you.

If you want to make moderate shifts to your eating plan to achieve balanced wellness, then you're a great candidate for this plan. On the macro diet, you are encouraged to set goals that promote balance and wellness. Restrictive eating practices and all of the symptoms that can result from severely cutting calories or cutting out food groups (such as constant cravings, an unhealthy preoccupation with food, and fatigue) should not happen on the macro diet if it is set up properly.

Anyone who has a strained relationship with food

The macro diet is also not a good plan for anyone who has a difficult relationship with eating. For example, if you identify certain foods as "good" or "bad" in order to plan meals or make food choices, then this diet probably won't be healthy for you. On the macro diet, any food is okay to eat, so nothing is "good" or "bad." Adding the pressure of reaching certain targets to an already difficult relationship with food may not be mentally healthy.

TIP

If you often have feelings of guilt or shame after eating certain foods and if those emotions have had a negative impact on your well-being, then tracking nutrients to meet certain targets may not work well for you.

Some studies have suggested that using diet and fitness apps or tracking apps that promote the quantification of diet (such as tracking macros or calories) can be detrimental to people who don't have a healthy relationship with food.

Anyone with (or at risk for) an eating disorder

The macro diet, or just tracking your macro intake, particularly with the use of a tracking app, can sometimes do more harm than good, especially if there is any possibility that you have an eating disorder.

WARNING

If you have an eating disorder, have a history of an eating disorder, or are at risk for an eating disorder, you should not pursue the macro diet.

Research has suggested that the use of calorie trackers can manifest higher levels of eating concern and unhealthy dietary restraint in certain populations (such as college-aged women). In some cases, the trackers may trigger, maintain, or exacerbate eating disorder symptoms.

If you are not sure if you have or are at risk for an eating disorder, online resources can help. For instance, the National Alliance for Eating Disorders lists these signs that may indicate that you have an eating disorder:

>> Hoarding and stashing food

>> Low body image

>> Low self-esteem

>> Obsessing over physical characteristics

>> Refusal to eat around others

>> Ritualistic eating habits

>> Struggling to engage with food in healthful ways

You can also visit the website of the National Eating Disorders Association (NEDA. org). The organization provides a screening tool (https://www.nationaleating disorders.org/screening-tool) that can help you determine if you are engaging in eating behaviors that may be interfering with your health.

WARNING

If you do find that you have or may have an eating disorder, you should reach out to a behavioral health expert who specializes in this type of condition to get care.

While the macro diet does help you to consume a more healthy and balanced diet, it also puts your attention on food and the quantification of food, which may not be healthy for those at risk for any type of disordered eating.

REMEMBER

No nutrition or fitness goal is worth compromising your health. If you have any concerns about your relationship with food, take some time to step back and get the care you need before trying this diet or any other.

Weighing the Pros and Cons

Before making a final decision to invest your time and energy in the macro diet, it can be helpful to evaluate the pros and cons. But remember, on the macro diet, you are in the driver's seat. You can experience the benefits without dealing with the drawbacks! But it is up to you to invest the time and energy into making the best food and meal choices to reach your goals.

In this section, I give you a rundown of the basic advantages and disadvantages so you can make the best decision for you.

Pros: Proceeding with balanced eating

The primary advantages of the macro diet will vary a bit from person to person. Your goals, your expectations, and the way you follow the program will impact these benefits. And a pro for one person might be a con for another. But you can scan this list to make a better decision for yourself.

>> **Maximizes flexibility:** In Chapter 3, I explain how you can make very gradual shifts to your eating habits when you start the macro diet. And since no foods are off limits, you can continue to eat the foods you enjoy, with (potentially) some adjustments to the amount you consume or other meals throughout the day. You can also go on or off this eating program as you see fit. Very few diets afford this level of flexibility, so it is easy to make it work for almost any type of eater in almost any kind of lifestyle and for any type of goal.

>> **Better diet quality:** No matter what foods you eat, you are likely to improve your diet quality with a macro tracking plan. Even if you consume less nutritious foods before starting the program and continue to consume less nutritious foods after starting the diet, just balancing your macronutrients will

be an improvement. However, most people find that they make better food choices when they start to prioritize nutrition.

>> **Budget-friendly:** Most people would agree that planning meals in advance helps to keep your food budget on track. If you plan meals around seasonal foods or products that are on sale, you'll save even more. Buying in bulk and cooking at home are also proven money-savers.

>> **Based on solid nutritional science and guidelines:** You don't have to follow nutritional guidelines when you go on the macro diet. However, I highly recommend that you consume protein, fat, and carbohydrates according to the advice provided by nutritional experts and organizations. I go into great detail about those guidelines in Chapter 6. The decision is ultimately up to you, but if you follow recommended guidelines, you are more likely to see the benefits I outline in Chapter 3.

Cons: Rethinking the macro approach

So, what are the downsides to this eating plan? There aren't many. But there are a few, and it is important to familiarize yourself with them so that your decision to start the diet is a realistic one.

>> **Can be time-consuming:** The biggest criticism of the macro diet is that planning and prepping meals can take a lot of time. Also, in the very beginning of the diet, you'll need to spend time setting goals and doing the math to find your optimal macro targets. On a day-to-day basis, you also need to take a few minutes to track the food you consume. But when you get a routine in place, the time you need to invest will diminish.

>> **Can be monotonous:** If you are used to eating something different every day for lunch and every night for dinner, then eating prepped meals (that are usually the same day to day) can be monotonous. If this is a concern for you, there are a few ways to get around it, like using different spices. If you prep meals to keep in the freezer, you'll be able to store them for a longer period of time. That allows you to pick from several different options when it is time to eat (assuming that you prepped several different types of meals).

>> **No guarantee of optimal nutrition.** When you compare the macro diet to well-respected diets (such as the Mediterranean diet), it *can* measure up nutritionally, but it completely depends on the food choices you make. A diet full of less nutritious foods that are balanced in macros is more healthy than one that is not, but in a perfect world, you want balanced macro and nutritious food choices to go hand in hand.

Tips to Help You Decide

If you are on the fence about the macro diet, these tips can help you come to a final decision.

Talk to others

If you know someone else who uses the macro diet, chat with them about their experience. However, remember that your experience may be very different than their experience if your goals, your needs, and your lifestyle are different. Still, your friend may be able to answer any questions and fill you in on the challenges and benefits they experienced.

You can also check out social media sites. However, if you are going to check sites like Instagram or TikTok, take the information they provide with a grain of salt.

WARNING

Some social media influencers might post insightful comments, but sometimes they also post images that are unrealistic. These images can be misleading about the potential results of the diet.

In some cases, the images show people who do much more than just follow the macro diet to get their results. In some cases, the images may be photoshopped or enhanced with lighting or other effects.

Evaluate your current goals and your goal history

Think about what you hope to accomplish with the macro diet. Have you set a similar goal in the past? What method did you use to accomplish that goal in the past? Were you successful?

TIP

If you've set a similar goal several times in the past and were unsuccessful at reaching it, you may want to adjust your new goal to avoid another disappointment.

Perhaps it would make sense to dial it back a bit and set a smaller goal that is more achievable. If you reach that goal, then revisit your original goal and decide if you are ready to take it on.

For example, maybe you have set a goal to get back in shape, and you are going to use the macro diet to help you improve your body composition. Your goal is to exercise every day for at least one hour. You've set this goal several times, but you always quit after a few weeks. Clearly, this goal is not realistic or sustainable.

Instead, you could set a goal to exercise three times per week to start. Then commit to spending at least two of your non-exercise days on macro diet meal prep activities (finding recipes, shopping for food, prepping meals). The combination of diet and (attainable) workouts is more likely to be sustainable and deliver results that last. If you are successful at this first phase, ramp it up just a bit for the next phase.

Examine your diet history

Have you tried multiple diets over the years without success? Were the diets overly restrictive?

For example, maybe you have set a goal to lose 20 pounds several times in the past with a calorie-counting diet but have been unsuccessful after repeated attempts. A more achievable goal might be to eat at least five servings of fruits and vegetables per day.

Macro diet meal prep can help you to achieve this goal. And replacing high-calorie foods with lower-calorie fruits and veggies can also promote healthy weight loss.

Try tackling this smaller goal first, then decide if you'd like to set a more substantial (but realistic!) weight-loss goal — such as one pound per week for two months. This type of step-by-step approach is especially helpful if you've had repeated unsuccessful attempts at weight loss in the past.

Track your nutrient intake for a week

Not sure that the macro diet will make a difference? Try tracking your current diet for at least seven days. First, you'll get to experience how tracking feels and which tracking apps work best for you. Also, you can get a handle on how your current nutritional habits compare to recommended guidelines.

You may find that you already eat a diet that meets the guidance offered by nutritional experts. Congratulations! In that case, you may enjoy the meal prep aspect of macro tracking, or you may give the entire diet a pass.

When most people track their current diet, they often find that they fall short (or go way over) in one or two macronutrients. This may give you the incentive you need to start the macro diet. You might want to target just one of those nutrients when you first start on the eating plan. Read Chapter 2 to see which nutrient would make the most sense for you to change.

Try a mini macro diet

If you're not ready to go all-in, that's okay. Why not give it a try using a toned-down version of the macro diet?

Use basic USDA guidelines as your macro targets (you'll find those numbers in Chapter 6). Then, decide how many meals you'd like to target. If you are short on time, choose just one meal per day to prep and track.

TIP

You can use a tracking app if you'd like, but you can also just balance your meal according to the easy plate method I explain in Chapter 7.

See how it feels to focus on macronutrient balance when preparing and consuming meals. Think about how you feel after eating and in the hours before your next meal. Do your workouts feel stronger? Have your cravings diminished?

Noting the changes you experience on the mini macro diet may help you decide whether the eating plan is right for you. It can also help you set goals and form realistic expectations for yourself if you choose to take on the macro diet journey.

2

Tracking Your Macros

Aim for achievable goals to set a clear path to success.

Calculate your personalized macro numbers that serve your lifestyle, your plans, and your body.

Explore different ways to track your macros so that you can choose the best strategy for you.

Chapter **5**

Setting Goals for Success

One of the most important steps you'll take to set yourself on the path to success has nothing to do with protein, fat, or carbohydrates. It doesn't even have to do with nutrition. You don't have to track macros or measure portion sizes during this step. Hard to believe, right?

REMEMBER

Nutrition experts and researchers alike have found that the simple act of goal setting can make a real difference in your results. However, the way you set your goals and manage your goals matters.

Of course, you might be thinking that simply starting and sticking to the macro diet should be your primary goal. But if you take some time to think about *why* you are making a dietary change and what you hope to achieve with your new nutritional program, you provide yourself with a firm foundation on which to stand when daily life intervenes and threatens to throw you off course.

In this chapter, I explain the goal-setting process and walk you through the steps, including identifying your priorities and fine-tuning the specifics so your goal provides you a clear path to success. I show you why goals are so powerful and tell you about the different types of goals that might be helpful in your diet journey.

You may want to set aside 30 minutes or more for this activity. Most importantly, know that goals can be revised throughout your journey. So don't worry if you feel that your goal isn't quite perfect. If you set a goal that seems unmanageable after a few weeks, simply revisit this process and make adjustments as needed.

Why Goals Matter

It is common to want to skip the goal-setting process. It can seem detached from the action-oriented components of your new meal plan, like grocery shopping, choosing optimal foods, and preparing meals. But if you understand why goals matter and how they play a role in your journey, you'll feel more inspired to invest time in this important step.

Goals provide a road map

It might be helpful to think of your macro diet journey as a long car trip. Every car trip begins with a destination in mind. You need to know *where* you want to go and why this destination holds value for you. Otherwise, you won't be motivated to take the time to travel there in the first place.

Next, you'll need a road map to serve as a guide and ensure that you make it to your targeted spot. You refer back to your road map if you think you are lost. The road map can also help you break down the total distance into shorter segments to make the journey manageable.

REMEMBER

By setting goals for your macro diet journey, you provide yourself with a road map to a destination — or an achievement — that is important to you. Your goal can help to provide direction and keep you on course as you navigate your journey.

Goal-setting can also help you to break down an extended process into manageable segments. Small, short-term goals provide stepping stones to help you reach larger, longer-term goals.

Goals help boost motivation

In the same way that a road map helps you understand where you are in your travels, goals can give you that same "You Are Here" reassurance so you don't feel lost on your macro diet journey.

Making dietary changes to reach a specific health or fitness outcome can be a long, drawn-out process. Knowing that you are on track and exactly where you are supposed to be can help you to stay grounded and motivated.

REMEMBER

If you use your short-term goals as stepping stones, you can look back at any moment and see all your hard work and achievements lined up behind you. Having a sense of accomplishment can serve as a healthy reminder that you can stick with your plan and achieve your long-term goals.

Lastly, you can also use your "road map" to remind yourself of how far you've come. This benefit is especially helpful when fatigue sets in and you need a boost of confidence.

Goals can help identify challenges

As you design your road map for success, you will likely identify challenges ahead. But just like you would do on a car trip, you can prepare in advance so that those challenges are easily surmountable. For instance, if you know that your car trip will involve a snowy mountain pass, you can be sure to travel with snow tires and chains.

REMEMBER

On the path to reaching your long-term dietary goal, you will probably need to change certain behaviors and habits. For most of us, change is *hard*. But if you are clear about the changes that need to be made, you can create an action plan for success that guides you from where you are now to where you want to be.

For example, let's say you've set a long-term goal to lose 30 pounds. You've broken that goal into manageable 10-pound segments that you'll tackle one at a time. During each segment, you identify specific dietary changes that will lead to the results you desire. But as you create your short-term goals, you notice that you've got a vacation scheduled that could derail your best efforts to stick to your plan.

To stay on track, you might set a short-term goal for your vacation that allows you to enjoy your trip without undoing any of your hard work and accomplishments so far. For example, you might take a break from counting macros during vacation and instead use a more relaxed method to maintain a balanced diet (check Chapters 11 and 12 for ideas about maintaining the macro diet while traveling).

By addressing the challenge ahead and creating a specific short-term goal for your vacation, you set yourself up for success. You can enjoy your vacation but come home knowing that you stuck to your plan. You maintain a sense of pride and accomplishment simply by using goals as your guide.

Different Types of Macro Diet Goals

There are different reasons that you might choose to track your macros. While the macro diet can be helpful if you are trying to lose weight, the eating plan is also popular among those trying to tackle athletic goals or improve their health. So, your goal may be weight-related, fitness-related, or health-related.

Each type of goal requires a slightly different approach. Consider each of these common types of macro diet goals to decide which one will work best for you.

Weight-related goals

One of the most common reasons that people track their macros is to reach and maintain a healthy weight. For instance, you might use the macro diet to help with weight loss.

REMEMBER

To lose weight, you need to create a calorie deficit. That is, you need to consume fewer calories than you burn each day.

But you will likely find that tracking your macros is the best way to stay within your calorie target without feeling hungry, fatigued, or deprived.

A balanced and nutritious macro diet provides your body with a variety of high-quality nutrients. You consume carbohydrates for energy. Carbs help you to power through your workouts, slide through that late-day energy slump, and (if you choose your carbs wisely) provide filling fiber to help you feel full and satisfied hours after eating.

The protein and fat you consume also boost *satiety* (the feeling of fullness and satisfaction after eating) while providing the building blocks you need to maintain muscle mass and contribute to healthy cell maintenance.

Weight loss isn't the only change that you might want to make to your physique. Maybe you want to increase your weight to improve your health or build muscle. A balanced macro diet is even more important if healthy weight *gain* is your goal. Of course, you can put on weight quickly by consuming fatty meals, sugary sodas, and calorie-rich convenience foods. But consuming a balanced macro diet will help to ensure that you maintain good health and build or maintain muscle mass while you reach your new target weight.

REMEMBER

Although any calorie surplus can help you to put on weight, a smarter approach to weight gain is to consume an optimized balance of nutritious macronutrients and pair the eating plan with a targeted exercise program. That way, you increase your body weight while maintaining a healthy body composition.

Athletic or fitness goals

You might track your macros as part of an athletic training plan. Maybe you've decided to start running, or you've started lifting weights because you want to increase muscle mass. Of course, following the diet alone can't make you sprint faster or give you big biceps. But if you set a performance-related goal, you can use evidence-based guidelines to tailor your macros to get the nutrition you need to train well and maximize gains at the gym.

For instance, if you've set a goal to improve your cardiovascular fitness, you'll probably want to build your macro plan around carbs. Endurance athletes like runners and cyclists must ensure they get high-quality carbs to fuel long training sessions. Organizations like the International Society of Sports Nutrition (ISSN) provide specific recommendations regarding the amount to consume based on your body weight.

TIP

The ISSN recommends that healthy exercising adults and individuals who participate in strenuous cardio activities consume 8–12 grams of carbohydrate per kilogram of body weight per day to ensure that they have the energy stores needed for training and competing.

Strength-trained athletes can also tailor their macro goals to maximize their training. Building muscle requires a focus on dietary protein. Protein helps to repair and build muscle tissue when paired with a regular strength-training program.

TIP

Weightlifters often increase their caloric intake and tailor their macro intake to ensure that they consume 1.6–2.2 grams of protein per kilogram of body weight per day.

Health goals

Counting macros can also help you to reach health or lifestyle-related goals. For instance, maybe you've decided that you want to get your blood sugar levels under control. You may be tired of the energy surges and slumps that take hold throughout the day. Or perhaps your healthcare provider or your genetics indicate that you are at risk for a health condition like diabetes.

TIP

If your goal is health-related, you may want to speak with your doctor or a registered dietitian to find out what a balanced macro diet can do for you. Can you reduce your dependence on medication? Or maybe a balanced diet can help you to get better test results. These incentives can help boost motivation.

You'll also want to know if specific macro targets are associated with the health outcome you desire. Gathering this information during the goal-setting stage will give you clarity as you move through the diet process.

Setting a SMART Goal

Whether your inspiration is performance-related, weight-related, or health-related, you can increase your chances of success using the SMART goal strategy.

Each letter of the SMART acronym stands for a different feature of the goal.

>> **Specific:** What do you hope to achieve with your goal, and precisely what will success look like?

>> **Measurable:** How will you know when you've reached your goal? What methods will be used to track your progress?

>> **Attainable:** Is your goal realistic? Have you achieved this goal or come close to achieving it in the past? Do you have the skills and resources available to attain your goal?

>> **Relevant:** Why is this goal meaningful to you? What will change in your life when you achieve it?

>> **Time-bound:** How much time will it take to reach your milestone?

Remember, you can set more than one goal. If the goal you have in mind is broad, you can break it down into smaller goals so that it feels manageable.

Looking at a SMART goal example

Let's try an example so you can see how SMART goals work. Imagine that you've been feeling sluggish lately and you've noticed that your weight has increased. You know that your diet has changed and you've started consuming more fast food and processed convenience foods. You suspect that the weight gain and nutritional shift has made simple daily tasks harder to accomplish. You'd like to regain your vitality by getting back to the dietary habits (and hopefully the weight) that you maintained for most of your life.

Now let's turn this into a SMART goal.

>> **Specific:** You know that the last time you felt strong and vital was two years ago when you ate balanced meals that were cooked at home. At that time you ate at fast food restaurants no more than once per month. So your goal is to gradually replace fast food meals with home-prepped food so that you eat fast food no more than once per month. You hope to regain your energy and lose the five pounds you gained as a result of this change.

>> **Measurable:** To monitor your progress each week you will track the number of meals you eat or prepare at home versus the number of fast food or convenience meals you consume. You also plan to keep a journal to track changes in your energy levels and weigh yourself weekly to see how your nutritional changes affect your weight.

>> **Attainable:** You were at your optimal energy level and goal weight two years ago and maintained that status in good health for several years. So, you know that your targets are realistic and healthy.

>> **Relevant:** Since your daily activities have been affected by the change in your diet, you look forward to "feeling like yourself" again and resuming activities that you've given up due to changes in your health.

>> **Time-bound:** You know that it will take some time to shift from a fast-food diet to a home-prepped diet. You also know that it takes time to restore your energy levels and lose weight. So, you decide to give yourself eight weeks to reach your goal.

This SMART goal addresses what you want to achieve and why it matters to you. These features help you to stay motivated as you move along in the process. But this goal is also fairly broad — it covers dietary changes, weight loss, and energy levels, and you'll notice that it doesn't necessarily address specifically how you will implement changes to make meals at home.

To refine your goal further and provide more direction for your process, you can set smaller SMART goals to use as stepping stones.

For example, you can set individual SMART goals to

>> Implement meal planning strategies and set aside time on Sundays to prep meals for the coming week

>> Research and stock your refrigerator with nutrient-rich snacks to boost energy

>> Add fiber-rich carbohydrates to each meal to reduce hunger and cravings

>> Walk 30 minutes each day to restore activity levels

>> Drink eight ounces of water with each meal instead of soda to optimize hydration

Each of these mini goals can give you a more specific focus. If your primary SMART goal feels overwhelming, focus on one of these for a short period of time. That way you don't have to make too many changes at once.

Tackling small goals one at a time makes the whole SMART goal process more manageable and increases the chance that you'll stay on track.

And, as you tick off each goal, you build confidence in your abilities to achieve your larger goal.

Succeeding with SMART goals

It will probably take more time to set your first SMART goal than subsequent goals. So, don't get discouraged if the process seems tedious at first. Once you get the hang of it, you'll be using the technique regularly — even in areas of your life unrelated to diet and nutrition.

You can do a few things to make the process more successful:

>> **Write out your goals.** Just thinking about your goals is helpful, but writing them out makes them more official. Create a document on your computer and print it out. Or go old school and use paper and pen. Some people even go a step further and create an entire vision board that includes their goal and images that they find inspiring.

>> **Post your document.** Once your goal is defined and written out, post it in a place where you see it regularly. Put it on your refrigerator, over your desk at work, or in your bathroom so you see it first thing in the morning. Having a regular reminder of your goal will help to keep you motivated and on track.

>> **Use social media.** If you are active on Facebook, Instagram, or TikTok, use the power of social media to hold yourself accountable. Let others know that you have set a goal and give them updates on your progress.

Revisit your goal and make adjustments as needed. Fine-tuning is an important part of the process so don't feel bad if you didn't reach the goal you first established. It simply means that the goal needs some tweaking.

If you revisit your goal and found that you've been successful, give yourself credit! Brag about it to loved ones, pat yourself on the back, or give yourself a reward. When you give yourself credit, you build confidence that helps to keep you on track and increases your chances of success with future goals.

Chapter **6**

Finding Your Optimal Macro Numbers

The key to success on the macro diet is finding and reaching your optimal macro numbers. That is, you want to find the right proportion of protein, carbohydrate, and fat that works best for *your* body.

It's important that these numbers are personalized. You might have friends or acquaintances who track their macros. They might share their numbers in casual conversations or post them on social media. But just because your super-fit coworker consumes 250 grams of protein every day doesn't mean that you should.

Every "body" has unique needs. Your numbers should be based on your age, body size, activity level, and goals. In this chapter, I show you how to identify your personalized targets. With your numbers in mind, you can more effectively reach your health, fitness, or nutrition goals.

TIP

You'll need to do a little bit of calculating during this stage of the process. If you're like me, you try to avoid doing math at all costs. But don't worry! This math is fairly simple. Or you can use one of the online calculators I recommend.

Are you ready to get started? This chapter walks you through the four steps to finding your optimal macro numbers. First, you find out how much energy (calories) you need each day. Then you decide how many of those calories should come from protein, from carbs, and from fat. Then you translate those ratios into manageable targets, and finally, you use those targets to decide how much food to eat each day.

Step One: Determine Your Caloric Needs

Calories provide your body with energy. The term "calorie" is generally used interchangeably with "kcal" or "kilocalorie" even though technically a kilocalorie (large calorie) is equivalent to 1,000 (small) calories. But small calories are too tiny to use as a measurement in nutritional settings, so the general term "calorie" or "kcal" is used (even on nutritional labels).

Calories are units of heat. One kcal is the amount of heat or energy needed to increase the temperature of one gram of water by one degree Celsius. You don't need to worry about heat and water, however. But it is helpful to remember that calories provide energy.

REMEMBER

The amount of energy that you need depends on your sex, height and weight, age, and activity level. Once you determine your daily caloric intake, you'll adjust that number based on your desire to lose, gain, or maintain body weight.

In clinical settings, your daily energy "cost" is referred to as your *total daily energy expenditure* (TDEE) and expressed as a number of calories. The four different components that determine your TDEE include

>> **Resting metabolic rate** (RMR): Calories necessary for basic bodily functions when your body is at rest, including the energy needed for basic physical functions like breathing and circulation. RMR is the largest component of TDEE and usually accounts for about 60–70 percent of your total daily calorie needs.

>> **Non-exercise activity thermogenesis** (NEAT): Calories needed for all of your non-exercise movements, including activities like cleaning and cooking. NEAT can account for about 15 percent of TDEE in sedentary people but can contribute up to 50 percent of TDEE in those who are very active.

>> **Exercise activity thermogenesis** (EAT): Calories necessary for exercise. EAT can account for roughly 15–30 percent of TDEE in people who work out.

>> **Thermic effect of food** (TEF): Calories needed to digest food. TEF generally accounts for about 10–15 percent of your total TDEE.

Don't worry. You don't have to come up with numbers for each of these categories. They are listed here just so that you understand how your body uses energy (calories) each day. Tests to determine TDEE are available.

WARNING

For example, many gyms and health clubs offer metabolic testing to help you estimate your RMR so that you can calculate your total daily energy needs. But the tests are often unreliable and can be expensive.

TECHNICAL STUFF

Some labs estimate TDEE using a procedure called *doubly labeled water* (DLW). The test involves a urine analysis after a tester drinks two different types of water. DLW is considered a gold standard for measuring TDEE, but it is expensive and not available in all areas.

So how do you get your TDEE number if tests are not an option? You can calculate your number using the Mifflin St. Jeor equation, a tool commonly used to estimate resting metabolic rate, including by organizations such as the National Institutes of Health. Alternatively, you can just use an online calculator.

TIP

Visit the National Institutes of Health Body Weight Planner and use their online calculator at https://www.niddk.nih.gov/bwp to get an estimate of the number of calories you need.

The Mifflin St. Jeor equation is slightly different for males and females:

Male:

$$(10 \times \text{weight in kg}) + (6.25 \times \text{height in cm}) - (5 \times \text{age in years}) + 5$$

Female:

$$(10 \times \text{weight in kg}) + (6.25 \times \text{height in cm}) - (5 \times \text{age in years}) - 161$$

After you get your number, you'll need to adjust it for your activity level. This is the last step of the process of calculating your daily calorie needs. Determine your activity level based on the categories shown in Table 6-1 and then multiply your number as indicated.

If you survived the math, congratulations! You're in the home stretch. You now have a science-based estimate of the total number of calories you burn each day, also called your TDEE.

After estimating your total daily energy expenditure (TDEE), you need to adjust your number based on your weight-related goals. Do you want to lose weight? Are you looking to gain weight? Or is your weight just fine as it is? You'll make a different adjustment based on your answer.

TABLE 6-1

Activity Level Categories

Category	Description	Multiply by
Sedentary	Little to no exercise	1.2
Light activity	Easy exercise 1–3 days per week	1.375
Moderate activity	Moderate exercise 3–5 days week	1.55
Very active	Hard exercise 6–7 days per week	1.725
Extra active	Vigorous exercise and a physically active job	1.9

Adjusting TDEE for weight loss

Are you ready to slim down? If your goal is to lose weight, you need to consume fewer calories than your body burns each day. When you do so, your body uses stored fat as fuel, resulting in weight loss.

REMEMBER

In general, experts advise that you cut about 500 calories per day for a healthy rate of weight loss. This number is based on the idea that a pound of fat is equal to roughly 3,500 calories. So, to lose one pound of fat per week, you should cut 500 calories per day for a weekly deficit of 3,500.

It is important to remember, however, that calorie estimates are just that: *estimates*. The belief that a pound of fat is equal to about 3,500 calories has been vigorously debated. But many nutrition and weight-loss professionals still rely on this number because it is the best estimate that we have to work with at this point.

Of course, you *can* cut more than 500 calories per day to lose weight faster. Crash diets often require that you cut 800–1000 calories per day. But going on a very low-calorie diet also increases the chance that the entire eating plan will backfire. It is also unhealthy, both mentally and physically.

WARNING

Severe calorie restriction often leads to fatigue and hunger. It can even lead to a strained relationship with food and disordered eating.

If you become hungry, tired, and stressed from a lack of calories (energy), you're not likely to last on the weight-loss program you've set up for yourself. In addition, you're not likely to get the vitamins and minerals your body needs to function properly. So, as you calculate your energy needs, cut no more than 500 calories per day unless your healthcare provider has suggested otherwise.

This example will help you to understand how the calculations work.

Imagine that you are a 35-year-old female who weighs 175 pounds (79 kg) and is 65 inches tall (165 cm). You have a sedentary job, and you do not exercise.

Using the Mifflin St. Jeor equation, you'll learn that you burn about 1,485 calories at rest. When you adjust for your activity level (sedentary), your TDEE is estimated to be about 1,782 calories. Subtract 500 calories for weight loss, and you are left with a daily calorie target of 1,282, which is fairly low. Keep in mind that you can always adjust your calorie adjustment to make your weight loss plan sustainable.

Adjusting TDEE for weight gain

Since weight loss requires a calorie deficit, it probably won't surprise you that weight gain requires a calorie *surplus*. That is, instead of consuming fewer calories than you need, you'll consume more calories than you need when you want to gain weight.

TIP

If you need to gain weight to recover from an illness, ask your doctor for a referral to a registered dietitian who can provide specific guidance to accommodate your medical condition.

A common reason for wanting to gain weight is to build muscle. In fact, strength-trained athletes often participate in a process called "bulking," in which calorie intake is increased (along with a more intense weightlifting schedule) to increase their muscle size, also called muscle hypertrophy. The bulking phase is usually followed by a "cutting" phase, where calories are decreased to lose fat and increase muscle definition.

REMEMBER

If your goal is muscle gain, experts generally advise increasing your calorie intake by about 15 percent, although some suggest a wider range of 10–20 percent. That means if you usually consume 2,000 calories per day, you might increase your calorie intake and consume 2,200–2,400 calories per day to gain weight.

You can also use your current weight to figure out how many calories to consume per day for weight gain. In a large research review published in the journal *Sports Medicine*, researchers found that bodybuilders consumed an average of 45 calories per kilogram of body weight per day during their bulking phase to gain about 0.25–0.5 percent of body weight per week.

It is important to remember that just because you eat more doesn't mean your body will naturally put on muscle. Unless you participate in a regular program of weight training, the excess calories will be stored as fat.

In fact, even with a well-designed bulking program, you are likely to put on some fat during this phase, which is why athletes often plan a cutting phase after they bulk up. During cutting, you might decrease your calorie intake by 300–500 calories per day. You don't want to cut too much, though, because you need calories to preserve the muscle mass you just worked so hard to gain.

For any muscle-building plan, calorie quality is important. You'll want to focus on protein so that you get the important amino acids you need to build and repair muscle tissue. (For more details about the amount of protein you need to build muscle mass, check out the following section.) Need to know more about the different types of protein? See Chapter 2. Shopping for protein powders? Let Chapter 14 be your guide.

REMEMBER

If bulking and cutting sounds interesting to you, keep in mind that it is not an exact science. Your best path to success is to work with a qualified sports nutritionist who can evaluate your progress over time and make personalized recommendations for you.

Adjusting TDEE for weight maintenance

If you are happy with your weight, then there is usually no reason to change your calorie intake. But you might want to reevaluate it every now and then.

Common reasons for reevaluating and readjusting your caloric intake include a change in your activity status, weight fluctuations, or frequent hunger.

For example, if you worked a construction job for many years, you probably burned significant calories from NEAT. Remember, those are calories burned with non-exercise movement, and NEAT calories can account for up to 50 percent of your TDEE. But if you recently took a desk job, you're not going to burn as many calories anymore. To maintain your weight, you'll need to decrease your caloric intake.

Frequent hunger is another sign that your TDEE needs to be reevaluated. If your eating pattern hasn't changed, but you find yourself hungry often, you can try increasing your calorie intake and see if the hunger subsides. You might also want to evaluate the type of calories that you consume. For instance, if you tend to eat a lot of starchy carbs, you might need to include more protein and fiber-rich foods in your diet to quell those hunger pangs. (Chapter 2 explains how different foods affect *satiety,* or the feeling of fullness.)

Fluctuations in weight can be another reason that you need to check your daily calorie intake. But this is an area where you need to exercise caution. Getting on the scale every day doesn't always provide an accurate assessment of your weight.

REMEMBER

Daily weight changes are completely normal. Your weight might fluctuate by five pounds or more from day to day due to water retention, hormonal changes, or other temporary factors. So, you don't want to make big changes to your calorie intake because you see a higher or lower number on the scale for just a day or two.

Instead, look for patterns. If your weight stays elevated or is lower than normal for several weeks, then consider making adjustments to your meal plan. Start with small changes (just 100 calories or so per day) and then make adjustments as needed.

If you continue to see weight loss or weight gain despite making changes to your food intake, speak with your healthcare provider. Some medical conditions and medications can play a role in your weight.

Step Two: Choose Your Personalized Macro Ratio

After you've established your personalized calorie target, then you can decide what portion of calories should be allocated to protein, carbs, and fat.

REMEMBER

The best ratio for you will depend on your health or fitness goals — whether you want to gain muscle, improve your cardiovascular endurance, lose weight, or simply maintain or improve your health.

You'll notice that most recommendations for macronutrient intake fall within the guidelines offered by major health organizations, such as the U.S. Department of Health and Human Services (HHS). A few diets severely restrict or eliminate certain macronutrients. The keto diet, for instance, substantially restricts carbs and reduces protein intake to emphasize fat. But remember, the purpose of the macro diet is to achieve balance. The macro diet is based on the belief that your body needs adequate amounts of protein, carbohydrates, and healthy fats to function at its best.

Macro ratios for general health

If you are at a healthy weight, but simply want to improve your diet to gain energy, feel better throughout the day, and optimize your overall wellness, you can follow guidelines provided by HHS and the U.S. Department of Agriculture (USDA).

Every five years these organizations assemble experts to evaluate recent nutritional research and make recommendations about what we should eat. They release the Dietary Guidelines for Americans (DGA), a document that provides detailed information for macronutrient and micronutrient intake, along with suggestions for healthier eating habits.

TECHNICAL STUFF

Unfortunately, most of us still don't follow the eating guidelines provided by the DGA. According to the USDA, the average American diet only scores 59 out of 100 on the Healthy Eating Index (HEI), even though research clearly shows that higher HEI scores can improve health.

Balancing your macros is a great first step if you want to follow the nutritional recommendations provided by the DGA.

REMEMBER

According to the 2020–2025 Dietary Guidelines for Americans, adults should consume:

>> 10–35 percent of your calories from protein

>> 45–65 percent of your calories from carbohydrates

>> 20–35 percent of your calories from fat (with only 10 percent or less of calories coming from saturated fat)

Since the DGA provides a range for each macro, you've got some wiggle room to personalize your diet. You can shoot for the ranges provided each day and aim to consume protein, fat, and carbs in the ratios suggested. Or you can dial the numbers down a bit to reach more specific targets.

If you prefer to use specific percentages (rather than ranges) for each macronutrient, then you'll want to fine-tune the numbers. To do so, you should base your new targets on your current macro intake so that whatever dietary changes you make are small and sustainable. Then make adjustments based on how you feel.

For example, perhaps you want to start tracking your macros to gain more energy each day. You've decided to use the DGA but prefer to have a more specific target for each macronutrient. The first thing you should do is track your current diet to get an idea of your macronutrient intake.

For one week, use an app like MyFitnessPal or another tracking tool (check out Chapter 7 to learn more about different tracking tools). At the end of each day, see what percent of calories came from protein, fat, and carbs. After a full week, you should see a pattern. Make small adjustments to your current intake to align with the DGA ranges.

For instance, let's say that before the macro diet, your intake of nutrients looks something like this:

>> Calories from protein: 10 percent
>> Calories from carbs: 40 percent
>> Calories from fat: 50 percent

To bring your intake amounts into alignment with DGA, simply make small changes to use as a starting point. So, your first macro diet targets might look like this:

>> Calories from protein: 20 percent (an increase of 10 percent)
>> Calories from carbs: 45 percent (an increase of 5 percent)
>> Calories from fat: 35 percent (a decrease of 15 percent)

You'll notice that each macronutrient target is now in line with DGA recommendations. But each number has only been adjusted minimally, so you don't need to make drastic changes to the way you eat.

After a few weeks, check in with yourself and see how you feel. Make adjustments to your plan and tweak your target numbers as needed to reach your goal. For instance, if you find that you are hungry often, you may want to dial back the carbs and increase your intake of protein and fat to help you feel more satisfied after eating. You might also try looking at the quality of carbs that you consume. Do they contain enough filling fiber? You'll learn more about how to monitor your progress and make changes in Chapter 9.

Macro ratios for athletes

If you work out regularly or compete in a sport, you can use the macro diet to support your training. Getting the right nutrients in the right amounts can help you to work out more efficiently and reach your goals. You'll have slightly different priorities depending on whether you participate primarily in endurance training or strength training.

>> **Endurance training** (or aerobic exercise) involves cardiovascular activities, like cycling or swimming. Walking workouts and elliptical workouts would also be considered aerobic training. Any sustained rhythmic movement that increases breathing and heart rate is considered aerobic or cardio training.

>> **Strength training** includes activities that build muscle, like weightlifting. Bodybuilders and powerlifters fall into this category.

TIP

Many athletes participate in both endurance and strength training workouts. To decide which category you fall into, determine where and how you spend most of your training hours.

TIP

If you don't have any specific goals in either category but you work out regularly and getting more fit is important to you, you can either follow the guidelines in the preceding section, "Macro ratios for general health" or use the "general fitness" guidelines in the following section.

Endurance athletes

Endurance athletes, like runners or cyclists, should prioritize carbohydrate intake. Organizations like the International Society of Sports Nutrition (ISSN) have underscored the importance of carbohydrate intake before, during, and after training and competition. So, if endurance fitness is your goal, you should figure out your carbohydrate needs first and then fill in protein and fat.

The ISSN makes specific carbohydrate recommendations for athletes at different levels. Instead of providing recommendations as a percent of total calories, they are expressed as grams per kilogram of body weight per day (g/kg/day).

If you are an endurance athlete, use Table 6-2 to figure out how many grams of carbohydrates you need per day. Write down your number and then jump to "Step Three: Calculate Macro Grams" to finalize your numbers for all three macros.

TABLE 6-2

Carb Intake Guidelines

Training Level	Carbs
General fitness (not training to meet a performance or competitive goal)	3–5 g/kg/day
Moderate training (2–3 hours per day of intense exercise performed 5–6 times per week)	5–8 g/kg/day
High volume training (3–6 hours per day of intense training in 1–2 daily workouts for 5–6 days per week)	8–10 g/kg/day

Strength-trained athletes

If you participate in a regular weight-training program and you want your meal plan to help you build muscle, then you'll build your macro diet around protein. Almost all guidelines for the amount of protein in the diet still fall in line with recommendations from the DGA.

The ISSN suggests that strength training athletes should consume at least 1.4–2.0 g/kg/day of protein to build and maintain muscle. But the organization also acknowledges that more than 3.0 g/kg/day may be needed for some weightlifters to optimize muscle mass and reduce body fat.

That's a pretty big range. So, the ISSN also suggests that about 1.6 g/kg/day is a good starting point. But if your current protein intake is significantly lower than that, you may want to start at 1.4 g/kg/day and gradually increase the amount of protein based on how you feel and how easy it is to reach your targets.

For example, if you start at 1.4 g/kg/day and can successfully reach that goal for two weeks, then increase to 1.6 g/kg/day and see how you do for another two weeks. Continue to increase in small increments until you hit your sweet spot.

When you've decided on a starting point, write it down and jump to "Step Three: Calculate Macro Grams" to determine specific grams and percentages for each macronutrient.

Macro ratios for weight loss

The best macronutrient ratio for weight loss is a highly debated topic. If you asked ten different nutrition experts for their recommendations, you are likely to get ten different answers. But what most will agree on is that the macro balance you choose should be sustainable.

When weight loss is your goal, scientific studies suggest that the best macro balance for you is the one you can stick to. But remember that maintaining good health is also essential, so the macro balance you choose should generally fall within the ranges suggested by the USDA for general health maintenance.

The USDA suggests the following macronutrient intake ratios:

» Calories from protein: 10–35 percent

» Calories from carbohydrates: 45–65 percent

» Calories from fat: 20–35 percent (with only 10 percent or fewer calories coming from saturated fat)

High protein diets have been shown to help maintain lean body mass (muscle) while also reducing body fat. Protein also helps you to feel fuller longer, which can be especially helpful when cutting calories. But you're probably wondering how much protein is best.

One well-known and widely used weight loss ratio is 40/30/30, a macro balance popularized by Dr. Barry Sears when he developed the Zone Diet. On this program, 40 percent of your calories come from carbohydrates, 30 percent from protein, and 30 percent from fat.

Although some scientific evidence supports this ratio for weight loss, it can be hard to maintain. And while the fat and protein intake fall in line with USDA guidelines, the carb intake is lower than recommended. The carb intake for the Zone Diet (40 percent) is lower than the intake suggested by the USDA (45–65 percent).

To find the best macro balance for weight loss, start with a ratio that is close to your current intake but one that also falls within USDA recommendations. You can focus on protein intake based on research suggesting that higher protein diets are generally more successful when trying to lose weight.

To determine your current intake, track your diet for one week. (See "Macro Ratios for General Health" for instructions.) Then make slight adjustments, prioritizing protein.

For example, you might track your diet and find out that you currently consume approximately:

>> Calories from protein: 10 percent

>> Calories from fat: 40 percent

>> Calories from carbs: 50 percent

Your carb consumption falls within USDA guidelines, so you don't need to make changes to your intake. But your protein intake is lower than recommended, and your fat is a little bit high. You don't want to make changes that are too drastic and unsustainable. So, you might try a macro balance that is manageable but also increases your protein intake.

Your new macro balance for weight loss might look like this:

>> Calories from protein: 25 percent

>> Calories from fat: 25 percent

>> Calories from carbs: 50 percent

This macro ratio for weight loss falls within the suggested guidelines but also bumps up the protein (at the expense of fat) so that you can maintain muscle mass while you lose body fat.

If this plan works for you, try bumping the protein up a little bit higher and reducing the fat or carbs based on your preferences.

TIP

Step Three: Calculate Macro Grams

You use ratios to set up the macro diet, but those ratios aren't terribly helpful when you're tracking macros on a daily basis. Even specific calorie numbers aren't very useful.

Since nutrition labels and tracking apps generally indicate the number of grams of each nutrient a particular food provides, it is easier to have your nutrient targets expressed in grams rather than calories or percentages.

Tracking grams rather than percentages also helps you to stay within your specific calorie targets. In this section, I show you how to get your numbers calculated.

This step of the process requires a bit of math. But don't worry, the calculations are simple, and you'll be a pro at it in no time. You'll use slightly different calculations for carb and protein versus fat.

Calculating carb and protein grams

All calories provide energy, but carbohydrates are the body's preferred energy source (see Chapter 2 for the lowdown on how carbs are used by your body). And protein helps your body to build and maintain muscle mass. So, reaching both your carbohydrate and protein targets is important for attaining health and wellness goals.

Each gram of carbohydrate and protein provides four calories. That means that one gram of carbohydrate is equal to four calories and one gram of protein is also equal to four calories.

REMEMBER

To figure out exactly how many grams of each nutrient you need, you'll first calculate the number of calories, then translate those calories into grams.

Say that you've determined that you need 2,000 calories per day to reach your wellness goals. You've also determined that your optimal macronutrient ratio is 30 percent protein, 50 percent carbs, and 20 percent fat. Now you can figure out how many calories of protein and carbohydrates to consume.

2,000 daily calories × 30% protein = 600 total daily calories from protein

600 calories / 4 calories per gram = 150 grams of protein per day

So now you know that your protein target is 150 grams per day. If you pick up a snack bar and the Nutrition Facts label indicates that a serving is one full bar and that serving contains 15 grams of protein, you'll know that you will meet 10 percent of your protein needs by eating that bar. If you were to consume two bars, you'd meet 30 percent of your daily protein needs.

Now do the math for the carbohydrate grams.

2,000 daily calories × 50% carbohydrate = 1,000 total daily calories from carbs

1,000 calories / 4 calories per gram = 250 grams of carbohydrate per day

So now you know that you need 250 grams of carbs each day. Perhaps along with your protein bar, you decide to enjoy a small banana. One small banana provides about 25 grams of carbohydrates or 10 percent of your daily intake, based on the math. (And, by the way, that banana also provides about a gram of protein, which will help you reach your protein target.)

A NOTE FOR ATHLETES

The ISSN provides recommendations expressed as a number of grams per kilogram of body weight per day (g/kg/day) rather than a percentage of daily calories. If you use these recommendations to determine your macros, your math will look a little bit different than the process that I describe in "Step Three: Calculate Macro Grams."

For example, imagine that you are a 180-pound (82 kg) weightlifter, and based on ISSN recommendations, you are going to try to consume 1.6 g/kg/day of protein. Based on your body size and activity level, you've estimated that you need 2,500 calories per day. First, you'll figure out how many grams of protein you need.

82 kilograms × 1.6 grams of protein = 131 grams of protein per day

131 grams of protein × 4 calories per gram = 524 calories from protein each day

524 calories / 2,500 total calories = 21 percent of daily calories should come from protein

Now you have a specific number of grams to target for your daily protein intake. And since you also have a percent of daily calories allotted for protein, you can fill in your desired targets for carbs and fat.

For instance, you might decide to consume 50 percent of your remaining calories from carbs and 29 percent from fat to stay within USDA-recommended guidelines. You can use the formulas for calculating grams of carbs and protein (explained in "Step Three: Calculate Macro Grams") to figure out how many grams of carbs and protein you should consume.

Calculating fat grams

We need fat to stay healthy. Fat also helps food taste good and helps us to feel satisfied after eating. But fat is more calorie dense than carbs or protein, so it is important to watch your intake, especially if weight loss is your goal.

REMEMBER

It doesn't matter if it is "good fat" or "bad fat," each gram of fat provides nine calories, more than twice the number of calories provided by carbs or protein.

To calculate the number of fat grams to consume each day, you can use the same process as you did for carbs and protein, but with different numbers.

If you need 2,000 calories per day and your optimal macronutrient ratio is 30 percent protein, 50 percent carbs, and 20 percent fat, you can figure out how many calories and grams of fat you need. The math would look like this:

2,000 daily calories × 20% fat = 400 total daily calories from fat

400 calories / 9 calories per gram = 44 grams of fat per day

Now remember that snack bar and banana example from the "Calculating carb and protein grams" section? Consider that scenario, but this time add two tablespoons of peanut butter and see how your numbers stack up.

Peanut butter is mostly fat but also provides some protein and some carbohydrates. You'll consume 16 grams of fat in that small serving, or 36 percent of your daily fat intake from the peanut butter. Those fat grams add up quickly! But that serving of peanut butter also provides about 8 grams of carbohydrates and 7 grams of protein to help you reach your other macro targets.

Step Four: Estimate Food Volume and Portion Sizes

When you start tracking your macros, you'll need to know how to ensure that the amount of food you consume delivers macronutrients in the quantities that you need. That is, you need to make sure you're getting the right amount of protein, carbs, and fat to reach your targets.

To figure that out, you'll probably use tools like a digital scale or measuring cups to portion out your food. (Chapter 8 explains how to use these and other important kitchen tools.) But it is also helpful to know how to estimate servings without special tools because you won't always have access to these gadgets, especially when you are eating away from home.

But first, it is important to clarify important terms related to food amounts. In casual settings, terms like "serving," "serving size," and "portion" might be used interchangeably. But they have very different meanings on food labels and in nutrition settings. You'll need to understand the correct meaning of each term to track food accurately.

REMEMBER

>> A **serving** of food is simply a measured amount of food, like one cup or three ounces.

>> **Serving size** on the Nutrition Facts label is the amount of food typically consumed in one sitting. This amount is determined according to U.S. Food and Drug Administration (FDA) standards. The FDA refers to this amount as the Reference Amount Customarily Consumed (RACC), and it is based on years of studying food behavior.

>> A **portion** of food is the amount of food that you choose to consume. It might be the same as the serving size, but it may also be more or less than the serving size indicated on the label.

The differences between these terms may not seem significant, but when you're tracking macros, it can make all the difference in the world. As an example, imagine that you buy a pre-packaged green smoothie at your local market. The label indicates that it contains 5 grams of protein per serving. So, you drink the entire smoothie and assume you've just consumed 5 grams of protein. Sounds simple, right?

But if the serving size indicated on the Nutrition Facts label is 1/2 bottle, then you've consumed 10 grams of protein by drinking the whole bottle. Your portion was twice the serving size indicated on the label. This is a common error made by new macro trackers. And while it can be a bit confusing in the beginning, getting the terms straight can save you from endless headaches down the line.

REMEMBER

The serving size indicated on the Nutrition Facts labels is not a *recommended* amount of food. You often assume that the amount listed on the food label is the amount of food that you "should" eat, but this is not true. The right amount of food for you is the amount that delivers the nutrients you need to satisfy your hunger and reach your targets.

You can look at different foods and learn how to estimate the amount of protein, fat, and carbohydrate that each serving delivers. Getting comfortable with these amounts can help you to reach your targets with less hassle each day.

What is a typical serving of protein?

Most macro trackers find protein to be the hardest macro target to reach. So, they prioritize protein foods when building meals and choosing snacks. You can use various techniques to estimate the amount of protein that different foods deliver. For example, you can use your hand or common household items to estimate the correct portion of various foods for you to consume. But remember that the serving size mentioned on food labels might be different than the amount you need or choose to consume (your portion).

For protein foods, like beef, chicken, or seafood, a typical serving size is generally 3–3.5 ounces or about 100 grams.

TIP

A three-ounce serving of protein foods is roughly comparable to the palm of your hand or a deck of cards.

It can be helpful to see how much protein you'll gain when you consume some of the most popular protein foods. The USDA provides estimates of the amount provided by a 100-gram serving of these foods. See these numbers listed in Table 6-3. You'll also see the typical or common amounts of each food that you might see packaged at the grocery store. Notice that the typical amount often varies from what is considered a serving size of each food.

Keep in mind that most of these foods provide more than just protein. When you eat them, you not only get closer to reaching your protein target, but they also provide fat and carbs to help you reach those nutrient targets as well.

What is a typical serving of carbohydrates?

Most of us don't have a hard time reaching our target for carbs. In fact, USDA data shows that Americans typically consume 34 teaspoons of sugar each day, which is equivalent to about 500 calories or 125 grams of carbohydrates. So, you might be reaching your carb target without consuming any nutrient-rich carbs that provide vitamins, minerals, and other healthy compounds.

TABLE 6-3   **USDA Protein Estimates**

Food	Protein per 100-gram serving	Common portions
Almonds	21.2g	One ounce of almonds (23 nuts) is about 28g, or 6g of protein.
Beef, ground (raw, 90% lean)	20g	A beef patty is usually about 113g, or 22g of protein.
Beef, tenderloin (raw)	20g	A steak is about 177g or 35g of protein.
Chicken breast (boneless, skinless, braised)	32g	A typical chicken breast is about 174 grams, or 56 grams of protein.
Cottage cheese (2% milkfat)	11g	One cup of cottage cheese is 220g, or 24g of protein.
Edamame (frozen)	11g	One cup of edamame is about 118g, or about 13g of protein.
Egg (hard boiled)	13g	One large egg is about 50g, or 6g of protein.
Lentils (boiled)	9g	One cup of lentils is about 198g, or about 18g of protein.
Salmon, sockeye (raw)	22g	A half salmon filet is about 198g, or 44g of protein.
Tofu (firm, raw)	17.3g	A quarter block of tofu is about 81g, or 14g of protein.
Tuna (canned in water, drained)	24g	A whole can of tuna is usually 172g, or 41g of protein.
Tuna, bluefin (fresh, raw)	24g	A small tuna steak is about 85g, or 20g of protein.
Turkey breast (sliced, prepackaged)	15g	One slice of deli turkey is about 16g, or about 2.5g of protein.

TECHNICAL STUFF

Many beverages provide carbs in the form of sugar. For example, a bottle of vanilla-flavored iced coffee provides about 36g of carbohydrates, and 34 of those carb grams are sugar. A 10-ounce "single-serve" bottle of 100 percent orange juice provides 32g of carbohydrates, and 25 of those grams are sugar.

To maximize health, you want to reach your target by consuming fiber-rich carbs, like whole grains, fruits, and vegetables along with some starchy foods.

TIP

To estimate serving sizes for carbohydrate foods, you can compare your food to common household items. For example, the typical serving size for cooked rice, pasta, or potato is about 1/2 cup or the size of a half baseball. A typical serving size for cereal is about one cup or the size of your fist. One serving of leafy greens is a cup or the size of a whole baseball, and a serving of fresh fruit is about 1/2 cup or a half baseball.

Table 6-4 shows USDA estimates for a 100-gram serving of common carbohydrate foods along with typical or common amounts of each food that you might find at your local grocery store.

TABLE 6-4 ## USDA Carbohydrate Estimates

Food	Carbs per 100-gram serving	Common portions
Apple	13g	One whole apple is about 216g or 28g of carbohydrate.
Banana	23g	One medium banana is about 118g or 27g of carbohydrate.
Beans, black (boiled)	24g	One cup of cooked black beans is about 172g or 41g of carbs.
Berries, mixed (frozen)	10g	One cup of mixed berries is about 150g or 15g of carbs.
Bread, whole wheat	43g	One slice of whole wheat bread is about 32g or 14g of carbohydrate.
Broccoli	6g	One cup of broccoli is about 76g or 5g of carbs.
Corn, whole kernels	26g	One cup of corn is about 141g or 37g of carbohydrate.
Pasta, whole wheat, cooked	32g	One cup of whole wheat spaghetti is about 151g or 48g of carbohydrate.
Potato, white, baked	21g	One medium russet potato is about 173g or 37g of carbohydrate.
Rice, brown, cooked	26g	One cup of cooked brown rice is about 202g or 52g of carbs.
Rice, white, cooked	21g	One cup of cooked white rice is about 174g or 37g of carbohydrate.
Sweet potato, cooked (no skin)	18g	One medium sweet potato is about 151g or 27g of carbs.

What is a typical serving of fat?

Tracking fat intake usually looks a little bit different than tracking protein or healthy carbohydrates. Fats are nutrient-dense, so a little goes a long way. Fat provides nine calories per gram, more than twice the number of calories provided by carbohydrates and protein. Because fatty foods are higher in calories, you're likely to reach your fat intake target without making a special effort to add fatty foods to your diet.

Oils used for cooking, marinades, salad dressings, and spreads all contribute substantial calories that add up quickly. Many dairy foods also provide fat. Be sure to include all of these foods in your tally when you add up your daily fat grams. It is also helpful to familiarize yourself with serving sizes for fat.

TIP

The serving size for fat is often considered to be one teaspoon, which is about the size of your thumb. But many foods that contain fat are consumed in larger amounts.

Each of the foods listed in Table 6-5 provides fat. Some also provide protein or carbs along with other important nutrients, like calcium.

TABLE 6-5   **USDA Estimates for Fat**

Food	Fat per serving	Common portions
Avocado	7g per 1/4 fruit	A whole avocado usually weighs about 200g, which is equivalent to 30g of fat.
Butter	4g per teaspoon	A tablespoon of butter is closer to 14g equivalent to 12g of fat.
Cheese, cheddar	9g per ounce	A typical slice of cheddar cheese is also about an ounce and provides 9g of fat.
Coconut oil	4.5g per teaspoon	A tablespoon of coconut oil is closer to 14g equivalent to 14g of fat.
Cream, half and half	2g per tablespoon	One ounce of half and half is about 30g or two tablespoons and almost 4g of fat.
Milk, whole	1g per ounce	One cup of whole milk is about 244g or 8g of fat.
Olive oil	5g per teaspoon	A tablespoon of olive oil is about 13.5g or 14g of fat.
Olives	7g per 100-gram serving (slightly less than a half cup)	Each jumbo olive (8g) provides just over a half gram of fat.

You might notice that the fat grams listed on the chart don't seem substantial. The problem is that fat is very easy to overconsume. If you are watching your fat intake, it's smart to measure cooking oils, dairy fats, and other fat sources to be sure you aren't consuming more than you need (and under-tracking your intake).

Chapter 7

Choosing the Best Macro Tracking Method for You

You can use dozens of different tools, tricks, and methods to track macronutrient consumption. What works best for one person may not be the best tracking method for another. So, it is smart to be aware of your options. That way, if you try one tool or app and it doesn't work well for you, you have other choices to experiment with.

You'll need to know how to understand and use different tracking aids, including the Nutrition Facts label found on all packaged foods, government websites, smartphone apps, and other handy tools and methods. But I've got you covered!

In this chapter, I tell you how to navigate the Nutrition Facts label so you can scan it quickly and gather essential information when you're shopping or preparing food. I also present you with different tracking tools so you can find one that fits your lifestyle and budget. This chapter also covers how different timing systems affect the macro diet so you can decide which one will work best for you.

Reading Nutrition Labels

Most packaged food items sold in the United States contain a Nutrition Facts label. The nutritional information provided on the label is supplied by the food's manufacturer, but the United States Food and Drug Administration (FDA) regulates the information that must be provided and the way it is displayed.

Canadian consumers will see a nutrition facts label very similar to the label found on American foods. In other countries, different systems are used.

TECHNICAL STUFF

For instance, the UK implements a traffic-light labeling system that uses color codes to indicate if a product is high (red), medium (yellow) or low (green) in fat, saturated fat, sugar, and salt. Some other European countries use a similar color-coded Nutri-Score to help consumers choose foods that fit their needs.

The Nutrition Facts label is updated occasionally to reflect changes to dietary recommendations. For example, in 2016 it was updated in part because increasing evidence linked added sugars to chronic diseases, such as obesity and heart disease. So, a line item was added to the label to indicate added sugars. According to the FDA, the updated label makes it easier for consumers to make better-informed food choices.

REMEMBER

On the macro diet, understanding how to navigate the Nutrition Facts label will not only help you to track your macros more effectively, but it can also help you to make the best food choices for your meal plan.

When you get comfortable finding and using the label, you'll be able to zip through the aisles of your market and make quick choices about which foods are best for you.

Key components of the nutrition label

Most Nutrition Facts labels follow the exact same format, although small packages can deviate from the format slightly due to size limitations. In that case, you'll find a label with a horizontal orientation, but it still contains all of the essential nutritional data in the same order as on the basic label displayed in Figure 7-1.

You'll notice that for each nutrient, the label indicates the number of grams per serving immediately to the right of the nutrient name. This is the number you want to pay attention to. Further to the right, you'll see a number listed under the heading "% Daily Value." Percent daily value tells you how much one serving of the food contributes to your total recommended intake of a given nutrient if you consume 2,000 calories per day. If you consume more or less than 2,000 calories per day, then the numbers won't be accurate for you.

Nutrition Facts

8 servings per container
Serving size   **2/3 cup (55g)**

Amount per serving
Calories   230

	% Daily Value*
Total Fat 8g	**10%**
Saturated Fat 1g	**5%**
Trans Fat 0g	
Cholesterol 0mg	**0%**
Sodium 160mg	**7%**
Total Carbohydrate 37g	**13%**
Dietary Fiber 4g	**14%**
Total Sugars 12g	
Includes 10g Added Sugars	**20%**
Protein 3g	
Vitamin D 2mcg	10%
Calcium 260mg	20%
Iron 8mg	45%
Potassium 240mg	6%

* The % Daily Value (DV) tells you how much a nutrient in a serving of food contributes to a daily diet. 2,000 calories a day is used for general nutrition advice.

FIGURE 7-1:
Nutrition
Facts Label.

© The U.S. Food & Drug Administration

REMEMBER

For the purposes of tracking your macros, you can ignore the percent daily value. Since you track your macros in grams, the number that matters most is the one listed in grams immediately to the right of the nutrient name. When you scan the label, be sure to look at these components:

>> **Serving Size:** The serving size is not necessarily the amount of food you *should* eat. It is the amount of food typically consumed during a single eating occasion. Instead of using this number to decide how much to eat, use it to determine how many calories are in a typical serving of that food. You'll also see the number of servings per container listed above serving size. Some food manufacturers even provide two columns of nutritional data, one for a single serving and one for the whole package.

>> **Calories:** This is the number of calories in a single serving of that food. In almost all cases, this number reflects the calories in the food as packaged, not as prepared. For example, a serving of pasta is usually about two ounces or 56 grams of uncooked, dry pasta. If you measure 56 grams of cooked pasta to

consume at mealtime, you'll end up eating less than a full serving because cooked pasta is heavier than dry pasta.

>> **Fat:** The total number of fat grams is listed first on the label; then underneath that, you'll also see saturated fat and trans fats listed. These items are on the label because the United States Department of Agriculture (USDA) has set recommendations for the intake of these two types of fat. Dietary guidelines suggest that no more than 10 percent of your total calories come from saturated fat. They also suggest that you consume as little trans fats as possible (although the FDA banned artificial trans fats, so it is less common to see significant numbers here). You might also see monounsaturated fats and polyunsaturated fats (commonly called "good" fats) listed here, but those numbers aren't required.

>> **Carbohydrate:** For the purposes of macro tracking, the main carbohydrate number (listed in grams) is what matters most. But for health reasons, you may want to examine the numbers listed beneath that number: fiber and added sugars.

REMEMBER

Fiber helps you to feel full and satisfied after eating. Diets higher in fiber have also been linked to a number of health benefits. So, choosing foods with fiber is smart.

Foods with added sugar have been linked to health problems. So, you may want to choose foods with less added sugar. And keep in mind that the number listed here is for *any* kind of sugar added during manufacturing. It doesn't matter if it is organic, or natural, or otherwise. Added sugar is added sugar.

>> **Protein:** The listing for grams of protein is at the bottom of the nutrient section, so it is easy to find. The majority of people on the macro diet will prioritize protein intake, so you want to make sure you check this number on foods you're considering.

>> **Vitamins and Minerals:** If you are trying to increase your intake of certain vitamins and minerals (called *micronutrients*), like calcium, or vitamin D, this is where you'll find information about the amount contained in one serving of food. Choosing foods with a wide range of micronutrients will help to boost overall health, which can help to make the macro diet more sustainable.

Need-to-know facts about the nutrition label

While the Nutrition Facts label is the most dependable and accessible source for nutrition data, keep in mind some issues when relying on the data for macro tracking.

First, the label isn't always accurate. Food manufacturers supply the nutrition data used in the label. But the FDA allows the calorie count of a food to exceed the calories shown on the label by up to 20 percent.

REMEMBER

Since calorie counts on food labels can be off by as much as 20 percent, the grams listed for each macro can be slightly off as well.

In one study of high-calorie snack foods, researchers suggested that inaccurate carbohydrate content and serving size were most likely to blame for calorie counts that were often higher than indicated. The potential for inaccuracy shouldn't deter you from using the numbers on the Nutrition Facts label, but it is helpful to keep in mind if you see discrepancies between numbers on similar products. Another potential accuracy issue involves consumer error.

REMEMBER

Consumers are typically bad at measuring serving sizes or remembering portion sizes. In fact, studies suggest that we often underestimate the amount of food that we consume, especially when it comes to less healthy processed foods and snack foods. This can affect the accuracy of macro tracking.

For example, you might choose to snack on a serving of almonds. The Nutrition Facts label tells you that the serving size is one ounce or about 28 almonds, and that is the portion you choose to consume. You're not likely to count your almonds before eating them, and if you don't have a scale handy, you're not likely to measure the ounces either. So, you estimate your portion and record the data for one ounce of almonds, which may or may not be accurate.

When you are first starting to track your macros, measure your portions as much as possible to get the most accurate data. You can measure your foods in many ways (explained in Chapter 8). But keep in mind that measuring doesn't need to be tedious. And you don't have to measure forever. After you get familiar with the serving sizes of different foods, you can start to estimate your portions.

Another concern regarding Nutrition Facts labels is that Nutrition labels are only required for packaged foods. So, if you eat a diet that primarily consists of whole foods, you won't be able to rely on the label for nutrient data.

For instance, you won't find Nutrition Facts labels on most fresh produce or on meat and seafood that you get directly from the butcher. You also won't find it if you buy grains, seeds, or nuts from the bulk section of your market. And if you buy local items from your local farmers market, you're not likely to find nutrition labels either.

REMEMBER

In many cases, the fresher the food, the less likely it is to carry a Nutrition Facts label. But that shouldn't deter you from choosing fresh whole foods. These foods are often more nutritious, and you can get nutrition data in other ways.

So how do you gather nutrition data when the label isn't available? Apps and websites provide information and can help you track your daily intake. The following section introduces you to a few different tracking tools so you can choose the tool that works best for you.

Using Different Tracking Tools

If you have a computer or a smartphone (or, more likely, both!), you'll have dozens of tracking apps and websites to choose from. But don't worry if you prefer to keep the tech tools out of the kitchen. There are old-school methods that work just as well. And if you don't like the idea of tracking, you *can* still follow the macro diet without tallying up your macros every day.

Consider all of the different methods listed here. You might find that the best tracking system for you is a combination of two or more tools.

Handy apps and websites

Nutrition apps and websites to help you gather and track macro information are numerous. The most popular by far is MyFitnessPal.

TIP

MyFitnessPal is the most widely used app for tracking macros. The smartphone app and website are both free and easy to use. You can also choose to upgrade to the premium level (for a fee) to get barcode scanning and other handy features.

But just because MyFitnessPal is popular doesn't mean it is necessarily the best tracking tool for you. Table 7-1 provides a list of different apps you can consider before deciding on your preferred method.

This isn't a complete list of every macro tracking app available, but it includes most of the popular options.

When choosing the best app for you, think about how you'll enter food into the system. For instance, if you eat primarily whole foods, then the barcode scanner may not be a useful feature because whole foods usually don't have a barcode sticker. If you eat out quite a bit, you'll want an app with a large database of restaurant foods. And if you cook, you'll want an app that has recipe tools.

Some websites are worth mentioning. For instance, one of the most comprehensive databases of foods — both packaged and fresh — is the USDA FoodData Central website (https://fdc.nal.usda.gov/).

TABLE 7-1   ## Popular Tracking Apps

App name	Fee	Description
Carb Manager	Free (with optional in-app purchases)	Designed primarily for people on the keto diet but can be used by anyone tracking their macros.
Cronometer	Free basic version with upgrades for an annual fee	Known for providing data from highly reputable sources such as NCCDB (Nutrition Coordinating Center Food & Nutrient Database) and USDA.
FoodNoms	Free basic version with optional upgrade to unlock more features	Allows you to scan barcodes for free and even scan nutrition labels. Provides a user-friendly, colorful interface that makes entering foods simple and even fun.
Lose It!	Free basic version with optional upgrade to unlock more features	Well-established, popular app that focuses on weight loss but can be used by anyone regardless of nutritional goal.
My Macros+	Small fee to download and then a monthly fee	Allows you to set goals that can be adjusted by a macro coach (with an upgrade). Barcode and nutrition label scanner are easy to use.
MyFitnessPal	Free basic version with option to upgrade for a fee	Easy to use and highly respected in nutrition community. Widely believed to have the largest food database, but it includes foods entered by users that may be less accurate. Also, barcode scanning only available to premium users.
Nutritionix Track	Free basic version with option to upgrade for a fee	Simple and easy to use website and app are widely used by nutrition pros, and the app provides ability to enter recipes and also includes a wide database of restaurant items.

TIP

The USDA's searchable site provides extensive nutrition data for foundational foods (like produce and meat) and for branded foods. Most entries also include a list of ingredients, which is helpful if you have an allergy or need to avoid certain foods. The data is updated regularly and even provides an update date so you know when the nutrition information was last checked.

Another helpful resource is Precision Nutrition (www.precisionnutrition.com). The site provides a wide array of nutritional information, including macro-tracking resources. One unique aspect of Precision Nutrition's macro tracking program is that they offer a plan that shows you how much food to eat using a hand portion system. For people who prefer not to measure or weigh foods, this is a great option.

Other sites, such as IIFYM.com or Macrosinc.net, provide macro calculators and some macro tracking resources. Each site has its own "personality" so you might want to explore a few if you want to use a website.

Old school journal method

Apps and websites make macro-tracking convenient for many people, but it is hard to knock the tried-and-true journal method, especially if you're a person who prefers to limit the amount of screen time in your life.

To track your macros with just paper and a pen, you can choose to keep a small notebook in your purse or briefcase so that it is handy when you eat a meal or snack. You can simply write down the food and portion size and fill in nutrient values later. Or, if you have time, you can fill in all of the data at the time of your meal.

TIP

If you use the pen-and-paper method, try to get at least the food and portion size jotted down as soon as possible after eating because we tend to be fairly inaccurate when it comes to dietary recall. Then you can fill in macro counts at the end of the day and tally up your numbers.

You can also use a template like the one provided in Figure 7-2. Make copies and post them at home or in your office.

You'll notice that Figure 7-2 includes space to write down each food and portion for breakfast, lunch, dinner, and snacks. You'll also find space to write down the number of grams for each macronutrient. The two columns on the right side of the table are customizable based on your needs. Perhaps you are keeping track of micronutrients that are important for your health. Or you can use it to track your alcohol calories. (Chapter 13 explains how alcohol calories are counted on the macro diet.)

TIP

If you use the provided template, be sure to fill in the date for each page and keep the pages when you are done with them. Keeping these records can help you to identify eating patterns or challenges that need to be addressed.

For instance, you might notice that have a harder time reaching your macro targets when you have important work or family obligations. If you notice a trend, think about ways to make your diet easier when your life gets hectic. Prepping meals in advance, for instance, is a great way to keep your macro diet on track when life becomes hectic.

Another trend you might notice is meal timing throughout the day. For instance, maybe you're great at consuming balanced meals in the morning and afternoon, but as nighttime approaches, you tend to crave sweet carb-rich foods. If that is the case, check out Chapter 17 for some macro-balanced sweet treat recipes.

DAILY FOOD LOG

Date_____

Meal	Food + Portion	Pro (g)	Carb (g)	Fat (g)		
Breakfast						
Lunch						
Dinner						
Snacks						
TOTALS						

FIGURE 7-2:
Daily Food Log.

CHAPTER 7 Choosing the Best Macro Tracking Method for You   105

Easy plate method

This method for tracking your macros is for those of you who aren't tech-savvy and prefer not to carry a notebook or keep a paper tally. In fact, it is the simplest tracking method, albeit the least accurate.

To do the plate method, you simply build your plate like you would build a pie chart using your macro balance as the general guide. The layout of your plate will look slightly different based on the macro balance on that you've chosen.

For example, if you've chosen to follow the general health guidelines provided by the USDA (see Chapter 6 for the ranges provided for each macro), you can follow the plate guide that they offer, called MyPlate. (See Figure 7-3.)

If you do choose to use this image as a guide, keep a few notes in mind. First, the plate sections are just approximations of how your food should be divided. There is no need to be exact in the way you plate your food.

Also, you'll notice on the image that there is a space (top right) for dairy products, which are not accounted for separately on the macro diet. Dairy products may contain all three macros (protein, carbs, and fat) so you can use this part of the image to remind yourself to consume dairy (if you include it in your diet) or you can ignore it and count your dairy intake as you would any other macro.

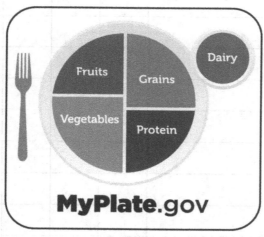

© USDA

FIGURE 7-3:
USDA MyPlate.

If your macro balance is 40/30/30, your plate would look very similar to the USDA MyPlate, but you'd increase your protein space and slightly decrease your carb space. (See Figure 7-4.)

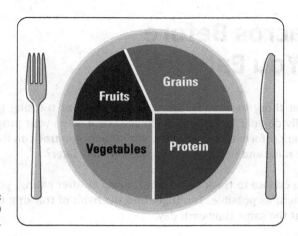

FIGURE 7-4:
40/30/30
Sample Plate.

The bottom line is that you fill each section of your plate with foods that fall into that macro category. Put lean meats, seafood, or plant-based protein (soybeans, tofu) into the protein section. Then divide the carbs section into grains, produce, or starchy carbs — but try to get a balance of each. Fill up that area with leafy greens, colorful fruits or veggies, brown rice, quinoa, or your favorite grains of choice. You might also put a sweet potato or pasta in this area. The more variety you add to your plate, the more nutrients you're likely to gain.

REMEMBER

But what about fat? You'll notice that I didn't add a section for fat on the plate images. Reaching your fat target usually happens without making any special effort to consume fatty foods.

For instance, many healthy protein sources (like dairy foods and seafood) naturally provide fat. And when you prepare your foods, you're likely to add a bit of fat, like olive oil used for cooking, marinades, or salad dressings. Since fat is more calorie-dense than carbs and protein, a small amount generally provides significant calories.

**TECHNICAL
STUFF**

The only macro dieters who may need to add a fat section are those who follow a keto diet. In that case, most of your calories come from fat, so you need to make a special effort to include fatty foods (that are also very low in carbs and relatively low in protein) to your plate.

Recording Macros Before versus After You Eat

An important thing to consider when setting up your tracking method is *when* you'll actually do your tracking. Should you write down your proposed meal and gather nutrient information before you eat? Should you track on the go? Or should you eat your meal and write down the nutrient data later?

TIP

Whether you choose to track before your meals or after eating, you should try to be as consistent as possible. You'll get into the habit of tracking more effectively if you do it at the same time each day.

Both timing strategies offer pros and cons. The following sections give you the pros and cons of each method; you can choose the best method for you.

Tracking in advance

Many people use a tracking app to plan meals in advance. It requires some organization and scheduling, but the payoff is significant. You're much more likely to have the right foods on hand, consume the correct portions, and reach your nutrient targets with accuracy when you know what you are going to eat in advance. Certainly, tracking in advance seems like the way to go. But it might not work for you; carefully consider the pros and cons.

Pros

Tracking your macros in advance helps you to see how your nutrient balance will play out and allows you to make the necessary adjustments so you reach your macro and calorie goals with accuracy. This strategy is especially helpful for those just starting the macro diet and for those trying to lose weight.

For instance, you might plan your Monday meals on Sunday evening. You would input each food and portion size into the tracking tool and then see whether or not you reach your nutrient targets within your calorie goal. If you fall short in one area or exceed your targets in another, you can make adjustments as needed. For example, you might have to adjust portion sizes or add a food or two to reach your goals.

TIP

If pre-tracking your meals every evening doesn't work for you, try doing it just once a week. Many people on the macro diet do meal planning one day per week (usually Sunday, but you can choose a day that works for you). You can do weekly pre-planning with meal prep or without. Visit Chapter 18 to learn more about prepping meals in advance.

Tracking in advance also allows you to prep meals or stock your kitchen ahead of time to make sure that you have all the necessary ingredients on hand so you are fully prepared at mealtime.

The most significant benefit of tracking macros in advance, however, is that it helps you to avoid decision fatigue. *Decision fatigue* refers to the difficulty we face making smart choices as the day progresses due to the sheer number of decisions we face over the course of a day.

TECHNICAL STUFF

Social scientists have estimated that we make as many as 35,000 decisions in a day, including everything from what to wear to work to whether or not to exercise. As the day progresses, the mental energy required to make these choices begins to wear on us, and decision fatigue sets in. When that happens, it is typical for our judgment to get cloudy. But that's not all; decision fatigue can lead to negative emotions, procrastination, and impulsive behavior. As you might imagine, these symptoms can affect your food choices.

WARNING

In the context of macro tracking, making food decisions later in the day can become more difficult simply because we are mentally tired. Decision fatigue can cloud your judgment. You become more likely to just grab whatever is available instead of putting careful thought into your meal.

But if you've planned your meals and snacks in advance, those decisions are already made. Your meals may even be prepared and pre-portioned, making the decision process even easier. You can simply revert to auto-pilot and carry out the decisions you made earlier.

Cons

Tracking in advance requires forethought and organization. In fact, the macro diet is often called the meal plan for Type A eaters simply because it involves so much planning and calculation.

TIP

If you are not a highly-scheduled person, you might drive yourself nuts trying to adopt the practice of pre-planning your meals and pre-tracking your nutrients. And that's okay! If you try tracking in advance and you end up frustrated most of the time, let it go. There are other ways to be successful on this diet.

Another issue with tracking in advance is that it doesn't leave a lot of room for healthy intuitive eating practices. *Intuitive eating* is the practice of listening to your body's cues and making food choices based on what your body needs (see Chapter 1). Intuitive eating and the macro diet can seem like they are at odds with each other. But they don't have to be.

For almost everyone, there should be some wiggle room in the diet to listen and accommodate your body's needs regardless of your macro or calorie goals. When you schedule meals in advance — with the expectation that you will eat the meals as planned — you don't leave a lot of room for variation in your food intake.

WARNING

If you are a person who is hard on yourself, you might see any variation from your plan as a failure, which can lead to a difficult or strained relationship with food.

If you think that planning meals in advance will put too much pressure on yourself to eat the "right way" or the "wrong way" it might not be a healthy practice for you. But if you can remember that your food plan has the flexibility to accommodate your body's cues, then it is more likely to work.

REMEMBER

Always keep in mind that in order for any eating plan to work, it must be sustainable. If tracking in advance doesn't work, then don't do it. You can track after eating or whenever it is convenient for you.

Tracking on the go

If you prefer not to plan meals in advance, you can choose to track your macro intake at mealtime. Tracking on the go works for people who don't mind taking a minute or two while eating to input data, but it's not a good fit for those who don't have extra time during meals or prefer to focus on their meal.

The primary benefit of this method is that it doesn't require the foresight and planning that tracking in advance demands, but it's still more accurate than tracking after you eat at the end of the day.

TIP

If you get into the habit of pulling out your tracking app or journal before you start eating, your numbers will probably be far more precise than they would be if you wait until hours later and try to recall what and how much you consumed.

Another benefit of tracking at mealtime is that you can still make some adjustments if necessary. Tracking in advance gives you the greatest flexibility to change your macros and tweak your ratios, but you can still make slight changes when tracking on the go.

For example, if you are tracking your lunch macros and know that your breakfast was a little low on protein, you'll probably want an afternoon meal with a bit more protein. If you input your foods and find that you are still a little low, you might be able to increase your protein portion to get your numbers where you want them. Of course, this will be much easier if you eat at home. If you are eating your pre-packed lunch at work or eating in a restaurant, your options are going to be limited.

The main downside to tracking on the go is that it can be annoying or time-consuming at a time when you may just want to enjoy your food. For some people, it may take the joy out of eating. In addition, if you are eating with others, they may not appreciate you taking out your phone during a meal.

Tracking after you eat

Like tracking macros before you eat, tracking it all after you eat has its pros and cons. The most obvious benefit of tracking after you eat — usually at the end of the day — is that it requires no pre-planning or organization. However, if you didn't hit your targets, you don't have the opportunity to go back and make adjustments. Your only option at the end of the day would be to add macros, which would also mean that you add calories.

Put bluntly, tracking macros after you eat is easier. You simply have to set aside ten minutes or so at the end of your day to sit down, enter the foods that you consumed throughout the day, and tally up your numbers.

For instance, if you tally up your macros at the end of the day, you might see that you hit your carb target and calorie target, exceeded your fat target, but fell short on protein. You could consume a protein food before bed to get those numbers up (but then you'd exceed your calorie target and potentially your fat target if the protein food contains fat — and most of them do).

Keep in mind, however, that most of us do a poor job of remembering exactly what we ate and how much we consumed. So your tracking numbers may be a bit off.

REMEMBER

Because tracking your macros after eating is less accurate, it is better suited for those who have less stringent calorie goals or for people who choose to prioritize one macro, such as protein.

In the preceding example, the macro tracker might be a bodybuilder. In that case, hitting the protein target is a high priority because they need important amino acids to build and repair muscle tissue. Eating a protein food to reach their target makes sense, even if it means exceeding other macro targets. And exceeding a calorie target won't impact a bodybuilder like it would someone who is trying to lose weight. In fact, the bodybuilder often wants a calorie excess. So, in this scenario, tracking at the end of the day can be a smart choice.

But what if you're not an organized person, you don't like the idea of tracking in advance, and you do need to prioritize calories because your goal is to lose weight? You can still choose to track at the end of the day. Your numbers won't be as accurate as they would with pre-planning, but you can still reach your goals.

On the days when your numbers are off, you can simply use that day as a learning experience and make an effort to adjust your in the future. In fact, you might be able to increase the opportunities for intuitive eating practices.

Let's revisit the earlier example and imagine that you are not a bodybuilder. Instead, you are trying to lose weight. If you know that you fell short on protein but met most of your other targets, you can use this information when choosing food the next day. Remember, protein is one of the macros that increases satiety (the feeling of fullness). If you pay attention to your body's cues and find that hunger is an issue throughout the day, you can use those internal messages along with the data from the previous day's tally to increase your protein portions and meet your body's needs while also reaching your targets more accurately.

REMEMBER

Whichever tracking strategy you choose, remember to leave yourself some room for trial and error. Learning to track your macros isn't (and shouldn't be) an exact science. Try different tools and different timing schedules to see what works best with your lifestyle and your personality. Eventually, you'll settle into habits that work well for you.

3
Making the Macro Diet Work for You

Set up your kitchen to streamline the process of making nutritionally balanced macro meals.

Monitor your progress and make changes to stay on target with your goals.

Compare different meal plans to see what the macro diet might look like for you.

Chapter **8**

Planning for Success

U nlike many restrictive diets, the macro diet puts the focus on eating. Instead of avoiding certain foods or saying goodbye to the thought of gobbling up your favorite goodies, macro trackers often spend a lot of time enjoying all aspects of food, including choosing foods, preparing foods, and of course, eating delicious meals, snacks, and desserts. Most often, they do so by mastering the art of meal prep.

REMEMBER

Meal prep is the process of preparing three to seven days' worth of breakfast, lunch, or dinner in advance. Usually, the meals are planned with your macro targets in mind, so it is easier to reach your macro diet goals.

If you're checking out this chapter and you haven't figured out your macro numbers yet, that's okay. In fact, you don't even need to be on the macro diet to reap the rewards of meal prepping. Many busy people prepare food for several days in advance simply to streamline their lives. And by doing so, they are able to make more careful choices about the foods they want to include in their diet.

To be clear, however, you don't have to spend hours in the kitchen to be successful on the macro diet.

TIP

If you don't like to cook or if you feel that your kitchen skills are lacking, you can still make this diet plan work. In Chapter 16, I go over various alternatives to cooking and prepping meals if you know that it is not for you. But my suggestion is to give it a try. Getting proficient in the kitchen empowers you to have greater control over what you eat.

TIP

When you are first starting out with meal prep, target just one daily meal. Choose the meal where you are shortest on time and the most stressed. It might also be a meal that you are often tempted to skip. You gain the greatest benefit from meal prep if you have a balanced, healthy meal ready to go when you most need it.

In this chapter, I explain why weekly meal prep has become so popular among successful macro trackers. This chapter also helps you sort through the kitchen supplies and gadgets that can make your new nutritional plan easier to follow. I give you food lists that you can take with you to the grocery store, so you can fill your fridge and pantry with healthy foods that you enjoy. And lastly, I talk about nutrient timing so you can decide when to eat meals and snacks so that you feel energized all day long.

Prepping Meals for the Win

Meal prep is often considered the cornerstone of the macro diet. While organizing your meals in advance is not required on this nutritional plan, most people who start and stick to the diet will tell you that meal prep is the key to success.

What those experienced meal preppers might not tell you is that it takes a little bit of time to get organized and settle into a routine.

TIP

Give yourself a month or two to experiment with different meal prep strategies. During this trial-and-error period, take notes about what works and what doesn't. This will help you to refine your process.

There isn't just one way to practice meal prep. With a bit of experimentation, you'll be able to find the best plan for your schedule and your lifestyle.

How meal prep promotes success

If you've never done meal prep before — and especially if you don't consider yourself to be proficient in the kitchen — the idea of cooking a week's worth of meals in one afternoon might seem overwhelming. But trust me, you should give it a try. Consider these seven reasons that meal prep is a winning strategy for meeting your health and nutrition goals.

TIP

REMEMBER

>> **You'll enjoy a more consistent diet.** When you plan meals in advance using your macro numbers as a guide, your body is going to get more consistent nutrition from day to day. This can help you to identify patterns and make adjustments as needed. You'll save money. When you plan meals in advance, it becomes much easier to make a specific grocery list, including the quantities of food that you need for each meal.

Also, when you plan meals in advance, you can use recipes that take advantage of money-saving sales or coupons. Increasingly, large grocery chains are putting coupons and offers online so you can do a bit of research in advance to maximize your savings.

>> **Your stress levels will dwindle.** How often have you found yourself wondering what to make for dinner on your drive home from work? Just thinking about the meal can be exhausting and stressful — especially if you have a full house and dinnertime tends to be hectic. When you plan and prepare your meals in advance, you take some important decisions off your plate, leaving more room for you to focus on other important aspects of your life.

>> **You'll boost your confidence in the kitchen.** It is not uncommon for people to describe themselves as kitchen newbies when they start the macro diet. But with practice comes proficiency, and proficiency boosts confidence and kitchen confidence might also boost your overall wellness. You're likely to try new foods more often and you may even become less dependent on restaurant or delivery meals if you know that a meal you make will be more delicious and satisfying. Over time, these factors can increase the overall quality of your diet and your enjoyment of food.

>> **You'll enhance your weight-loss efforts.** Prepped meals provide predictable portions on a consistent basis. Furthermore, they can be set up to deliver the nutrients that specifically target hunger — like fiber, protein, and healthy fat. Also, when you prep meals in advance, you avoid making decisions when you are tired or hungry.

By prepping meals in advance, you avoid making decisions about what to eat and how much to eat in the heat of the moment when you're hungry, tired, or stressed. This can help you keep on track on days when your willpower is waning.

>> **You'll make your macro diet more efficient.** There's no doubt that the primary reason for meal prepping on the macro diet is simplicity and efficiency. When you plan meals in advance (even if it is just one meal per day), you do all of the nutritional calculations only once, and you do them in advance. So, as you navigate through your day, you have the confidence of knowing that your nutritional plan is on track without having to stop and do any calculations or math.

Time-saving strategies to make meal prep more effective

You can implement a few organizational strategies to streamline your meal-prep process. These hacks can also help you stay on track with the macro diet when you are tempted to bypass your meal plan. Of course, there is nothing wrong with listening to your body when you have a craving or feel that you prefer something different to eat. But the more you can stick with the targets you set for yourself, the more likely you are to reach your goals.

Set a schedule and stick to it!

Choose one or two days per week for meal prep. Try to choose days when you know you'll have a few hours to devote to shopping, prepping, and packaging meals. Then make the date a priority.

TIP

Schedule your meal prep activities just like you would schedule all of your other important appointments. Pen it into your calendar and set a reminder on your smartphone or tablet.

Get savvy at the grocery store

Go grocery shopping after your meals have been planned. Create a detailed list based on your recipes. The list should include not only the food you need but also the quantity. You can even organize your list by department (see the food lists in "Optimizing Food Choices for Better Health") to make shopping quicker and easier.

TIP

Have a snack before heading to the market (shopping on an empty stomach is never a good idea) and approach the store with a strategy in mind. For example, shop the freezer aisles last so that food doesn't thaw while you're shopping.

Organize your fridge with smart food choices in mind

Believe it or not, a clean organized fridge can help you to make healthier food choices. When nutritious foods are buried behind stacks of soda cans, half-empty condiment containers, and last week's leftovers, you're not likely to see them when it's time to eat. So, before you start meal prep, take an hour or so to clean out your fridge to optimize healthy choices.

First, remove everything and dump anything that is out of date. Then refill your fridge, leaving the middle shelves available for your healthy prepped meals and other nutritious snacks that you want to have on hand. Then when you open the refrigerator door, you'll see the best options first.

Create a designated food prep zone

If you share a kitchen, try to set aside an area of the kitchen where you can keep all of your food prep supplies. For instance, you might keep your meal prep essentials on a pantry shelf or in a cabinet below your counter. You might even want to designate a "safe space" in your refrigerator where only your prepped foods are stored.

REMEMBER

When you know where all of your supplies are, you'll save time during the food-prep process because you won't have to deal with the hassle of gathering supplies every week. You may even want to decorate your space with inspiring slogans or notes about your progress.

So, what supplies will you need for your designated food prep space? The following section explains which kitchen tools and gadgets you may want to have on hand.

Setting Up Your Kitchen

As meal prep and macro tracking have gotten more popular, the marketplace has become saturated with tools and gadgets to make meal prep easier. But you don't need to break the bank and buy dozens of supplies to make your diet a success. Some products are important, but others may not be necessary, especially when you are just starting out. As you scan the lists in this section, you can make decisions about where you want to invest and what tools are best for you.

TIP

Having a well-stocked, well-organized kitchen will make sticking to the macro diet much easier. You'll spend far less time prepping meals and far more time enjoying them if you have all the necessary tools and foods on hand to whip up delicious meals and treats.

In this section, I explain the different kitchen tools that you might use when preparing healthy meals. I've organized them in order of general necessity. Some of these products are essential; some are helpful but not absolutely necessary; and others are nice to have but definitely not required for success. That way, you can stock your kitchen according to your budget.

Essential tools

Many cooks will already have these tools in their kitchen. But if you usually don't prepare your own meals, you may need to grab some of these items. You use most of these tools to make or store recipes in this book.

>> **Blender or food processor:** This might be the most expensive essential home cooking tool on the list (although good knives can be pricey). Some high-end blenders cost hundreds or even thousands of dollars. But you don't need to break the bank to get a tool to make soups and smoothies. When you're first starting out, find a basic model that fits your budget. Then when you know how often you use the appliance, you'll have a better idea if spending more money on one makes sense. Consider size (a single-serve blender won't work well if you plan to make soup in large batches) and power (you'll want at least three settings) when you shop.

>> **Cutting boards:** A high-quality cutting board will help preserve the blade of your knives and can also make food prep cleaner and safer. You might consider wood, bamboo, or plastic boards. When choosing a board, you might want to look for one that is dishwasher safe and one that has non-skid feet. Some cooks prefer to have multiple boards, one for meat, one for veggies, and one for fish, to enhance food safety. They are often sold in sets.

>> **Digital scale:** A digital scale is the easiest way to measure food portions quickly and accurately. Look for a scale that has a "tare" button which allows you to zero out the scale with an empty container on top. That way you can set foods inside the container for easier weighing, but the weight of the container won't be included in the result. You will also want to look for a scale that can be cleaned easily as you will probably be weighing foods like poultry or seafood.

>> **Food storage containers:** You need resealable containers that have airtight lids to store bulk foods that you eat during the week, like shredded chicken, rice, or beans. Get at least two to five containers in a range of different sizes. Many grocery stores and home goods stores sell sets for a reasonable price. As an alternative, you can use mixing bowls and plastic wrap, but investing in dedicated containers will make food storage much easier.

>> **Measuring cups:** Most cooks have at least one set of measuring cups for dry goods (like flour or grains) and at least one measuring cup for liquids (like milk or oil). You *can* use them interchangeably, but the measurements won't be as precise. Since these items tend to be inexpensive, it's usually worth it to get both types. In fact, you may want to get a few sets of dry measuring cups. They can be handy to keep in cannisters of foods like cereal or grains that you

use in the same amount regularly. For instance, if you usually consume one cup of cereal in the morning, you can keep a one-cup scoop with the cereal so you always get a precise amount.

>> **Measuring spoons:** Most recipes require that you measure cooking oils, spices, and other ingredients. For those tasks, you want measuring spoons that come in various sizes (tablespoon, teaspoon, half teaspoon, and so forth). Also, some cooks look for spoons that are deep and narrow with long handles so they fit into small spice jars.

>> **Mixing bowls:** Meal prep often involves mixing large quantities of chopped veggies, meat, or grains. So, you'll want at least one large bowl. Medium and smaller bowls are handy for mixing dressings and seasonings. But you can also use a cereal bowl in a pinch for those tasks. Often, mixing bowls are sold in sets, so you can get one of each size. Glass bowls are handy because they are usually microwave and dishwasher-safe, but they are also heavy. So, some cooks choose metal, plastic, or silicone bowls instead.

>> **Non-stick skillet or sauté pan:** You'll use a stove-top skillet to sauté onions, veggies, or meat for many of your meals. A non-stick skillet makes cooking easier and helps you to control the amount of cooking oil that you use. A sauté pan and a skillet are technically two different pans, but you can usually use them interchangeably in basic cooking. A skillet has tall vertical sides, and a sauté pan has sides that flare outward slightly. You'll find endless options at various price points in cooking stores and online. When shopping, think about the weight of the pan, the handle (some handles get hot, and some don't), and the material (you may want one that is dishwasher safe). This is another item where you can invest a lot of money if you want to, but when you're first starting out, getting a basic tool is best until you get a better sense of your cooking style and preferences.

>> **Quality knives:** You want to have at least one good knife, but most savvy cooks have at least three. A paring knife (3") helps with tasks that require a delicate cut, like removing the core from a tomato. A chef's knife (8" or 10") has a wider blade and is used for chopping. Then finally, a serrated knife is helpful for cutting foods that have one texture on the outside and one texture on the inside — like a tomato or crusty bread. If you plan to purchase only one knife, the chef's knife is probably your best bet.

>> **Sheet pans:** When you roast veggies, meats, or seafood, a good sheet pan will help food cook evenly with less mess. But keep in mind that a sheet pan is not the same as a cookie sheet, even though they look similar. A sheet pan has a distinctive rim (usually about one inch) that helps to keep meat juices or small bits of food from rolling off the pan.

>> **Storage bags:** Resealable storage bags are helpful for items like chopped veggies, berries, or small servings of grains. It is helpful to get them in different sizes (quart size, gallon size, sandwich size, and snack size) for different types of food. For example, snack-sized baggies are great for single servings of berries or nuts. Gallon-sized freezer bags can be used to store larger quantities of chili or soup in the freezer. Most of the storage bags that you find in the grocery store are disposable, but environmentally-friendly, re-useable silicone bags also are available in some stores and online. Look for BPA-free bags if you have concerns about potential exposure to toxins.

Helpful tools

After you've gotten comfortable with the meal prep process, you'll be able to get a better sense of the tools and gadgets that are useful for you. These products are not must-haves, but they can make preparing, storing, and carrying healthy meals easier.

>> **Colander or strainer:** You'll probably include foods like canned beans, steamed or boiled veggies, and pasta in some of your regular meals. Therefore, having a drainage tool on hand is smart. A colander and a strainer are two different tools, but they can usually be used interchangeably. A strainer is a hand-held device with a bowl made from mesh, and a colander has "feet," so you can place it in the sink and safely drain hot foods like pasta. In a professional kitchen, they might be used differently, but at home, you can use either one for almost anything that requires draining or rinsing.

>> **Crockpot or slow cooker:** Many successful macro trackers swear by their Crockpot meals. Why? Nothing is more convenient than placing a few food items in your cooker in the morning, heading off to the gym or to work, and then coming home to a warm, delicious meal. Endless options for using this appliance exist, so it's a smart one to invest in. A Crockpot and a slow cooker are the same appliances; Crockpot is simply a popular brand name. The appliance comes in different sizes, so look for a larger one if you plan to cook multiple meals in it. You can spend $200 or more for this appliance, but you can also find them for far less.

>> **Food labels:** After you store your food in the refrigerator or pantry, it is helpful to have labels on the containers that remind you of the "best by" date or nutrition facts. Craft stores and online suppliers sell reusable, removable, and even dissolvable labels that can come in handy to help keep you organized.

>> **Grater:** When you're first starting to count your macros, it might be easiest to buy pre-grated cheese (or even vegetables). It is definitely a time-saver. But you might notice that pre-grated cheese doesn't melt as well as block cheese that you grate at home. That's because pre-grated cheese is usually coated with a preservative that keeps it from clumping together. A decent four-sided box grater gives you multiple options for grating and slicing at home, and you can usually find one for less than $20.

>> **Insulated lunch bag:** If you go to the office most days or plan to eat one of your meals away from home, an insulated lunch bag will allow you to carry your prepped meals safely when they contain perishable items. If you only plan to carry one meal at a time, you can find a simple, single-compartment bag for less than the cost of a hearty lunch at a fast-casual restaurant.

TIP

You can store the bag in the freezer the night before you use it and then pack and carry it the following day.

>> **Mason jars:** These glass containers are a fan favorite with people who enjoy overnight oats. While you can use different types of containers for this morning meal, mason jars provide a tight seal that helps to keep your oats fresh. Also, the glass jar is easy to put in the microwave when you're ready to eat.

>> **Meal-prep containers:** If you plan to eat away from home often, you may want to invest in specific meal-prep containers instead of using basic storage containers for your meal. Several types of containers have two, three, or four separate sections, allowing you to keep your meat, grains, and veggies separate. When choosing the best containers, look for those that are dishwasher-safe, microwave safe, clear, leak-proof, air-tight, and durable.

>> **Muffin tin:** Most bakers have this item in their kitchen already. It's nearly impossible to make cupcakes or muffins without one. But meal preppers use this pan to make a wider range of meals. You can use it to make mini-meatloaves, single-serving egg bites, veggie and grain bakes, and so much more. Metal muffin tins conduct heat well and are usually easy to clean (many have a non-stick coating).

Nice tools to have (but not required)

There is no shortage of gadgets designed for those who practice meal prepping. Sometimes these gadgets are more hype than help, but depending on your cooking preferences, you might find some of these products useful.

>> **Air fryer:** This wildly popular kitchen appliance "fries" your food without oil. Whether or not they are worth it is a matter of great debate. Some cooks feel

that they don't provide any significant advantage over the oven. And often, the capacity of the device is limited. But many cooks swear by their air fryers, pointing to the fact that they provide a crispy fried-like texture and plenty of taste without the oil. If you're a fan of fried foods, then this appliance might be right for you. But if you already enjoy roasted veggies and meats, then it might not be worth the investment.

>> **Baggie holders:** If you store much of your food in sandwich or snack-sized baggies, then you know it can be a hassle to hold the bags open when you have to fill many of them. Believe it or not, a product exists to solve this pesky problem. Often called "baggy racks," these gadgets are inexpensive and easily found online.

As an alternative, however, you can use a few drinking glasses. Simply place the bag inside the glass with the ends folded over the top to hold the bag open when filling.

>> **Food journal:** If meal prep becomes a way of life for you, a journal can come in handy when you want to save recipes with nutrition facts, notes about prepping, or time-saving tips. Some people store these notes online, but an old-school journal can be kept in a kitchen drawer and used to save all of your important information.

>> **Portion-control plates:** If your goal is weight loss, you might want to consider a set of portion-control plates. Many of them look very much like the MyPlate design I share in Chapter 7. The plate serves as a reminder of how a balanced meal should look and what a healthy portion of each macro might look like. While this tool is not a sure fire tool for success, some researchers (as recently as 2022) found that the plates can enhance the weight-loss process when included as part of a comprehensive plan.

>> **Rice cooker:** Many cooks, even those who have spent years in the kitchen, find that cooking rice is tricky. If the ratio of water and rice is not perfect, you can end up with a sticky mess. The solution? A rice cooker. A rice cooker prepares rice perfectly every single time. And that's not all; many home cooks prepare other types of grains in this device. If you decide to buy one, do your homework. The price range is significant, but even the least expensive models can set you back.

>> **Salad dressing containers:** If you take your meals on the go and they require dressing or sauce on the side, you'll want small tightly-sealed containers. That way, your salad doesn't get soggy before it is time to eat. While these are not expensive, they are also not entirely necessary. You can also put salad dressing or sauces in snack sized baggies (although if you don't seal them well, they might leak).

>> **Salad spinner or produce keeper:** A salad spinner is basically a colander housed inside a larger bowl with a spinning device attached so that you can

rinse your leafy greens, spin the bowl to get rid of excess moisture, and the water is trapped below the greens in the outer bowl. Some spinners are also handy for keeping produce fresh in the fridge. After you get used to meal prep, you'll learn the right quantity to buy so they don't go bad. But this type of device can be helpful for extending the life of your leafy greens by a day or so.

» **Smoothie shaker:** Many gym-goers pack a smoothie shaker with dry ingredients ready to blend for after a workout. For instance, they might add protein powder and peanut powder to their shaker and fill it with water or almond milk when they are ready for their shake. Most smoothie shakers are made from lightweight plastic and have an internal device to make blending more efficient. If you are particular about the type of protein powder you use and you consume smoothies regularly, this inexpensive device might come in handy.

» **Specialty chopping tools:** If you find chopping to be a tedious task, many gadgets are made just for you. Some products are made to chop foods like hard boiled eggs, onions, and other fruits and veggies. Most are fairly inexpensive, so you don't have to break the bank for this convenience.

» **Thermos:** You'll probably only need a thermos if you eat away from home regularly and you enjoy meals like soup or chili. Liquid foods won't store or carry well in any meal prep container, so your best bet is a device designed just for that type of meal. Again, a thermos won't break the bank, so it may be a worthwhile investment for you if you like soup. You can also pack meals like pasta dishes in a thermos if you'd like.

Optimizing Food Choices for Better Health

The meals you prep can only be as nutritious as the ingredients you choose to use. So, it is smart to get savvy about the foods you buy. Of course, any recipe will provide you with a list of ingredients that are required. But when you head to the grocery store, you'll probably have a few options regarding the brand and type of that food that you put in your cart.

TIP

Learning more about the language on food labels — both the front of the label and the Nutrition Facts on the back of the label — will help you to make better choices when you shop. And understanding various descriptions for fresh foods (like fresh meats, poultry, and seafood) can help you to save money while optimizing nutrition.

To learn more about the Nutrition Facts label (usually located on the back or side of the food packages), visit Chapter 7, where I go through each line item in detail. In this next section, I explain what other types of food claims mean on product packaging. These claims are usually seen on the front of the package. Then I provide suggestions for different types of protein, carbohydrates, and fats to use in your cooking.

Decoding food claims

Food manufacturers can make health or nutrition claims about their food, but they have to follow certain government guidelines established by the U.S. Food and Drug Administration (FDA). For example, you might imagine that any food labeled as "healthy" provides the best possible blend of quality nutrients. But that is not necessarily the case. In fact, the FDA has spent years trying to determine exactly what "healthy" should mean on a food label.

REMEMBER

According to the FDA, healthy on a food label means that the food stays within certain limits for total fat, saturated fat, cholesterol, and sodium. These limits vary based on the type of food. Also, to qualify, foods must provide at least 10 percent of the daily value (DV) for one or more of the following nutrients: vitamin A, vitamin C, calcium, iron, protein, and fiber.

As of September 2022, discussions were still ongoing about how and why this definition should be updated. For instance, many dietitians and nutrition experts feel that added sugars need to be considered when evaluating whether or not a food is healthy.

REMEMBER

For now, consumers should understand that front-of-package claims don't always mean what you think they mean. So always check the Nutrition Facts label to see if a food aligns with your personalized nutritional goals.

Let's break down some of the more popular claims and decode their specific meanings according to the FDA. Understanding the exact meaning of each description can help you to feel more empowered as you shop. Table 8-1 presents nutritional claims and their meanings as defined by the FDA.

Keep in mind that as you shop and read food packages, these claims don't mean that a particular product is necessarily "good" or necessarily "bad." They simply help you determine whether or not the food aligns with your nutritional goals.

TABLE 8-1

Claim	Definition
Calorie-free	Less than 5 calories per serving
Low in calories	Less than 40 calories per serving
Reduced-calorie	At least 25 percent fewer calories per serving than a comparable food
Fat-free	Less than 0.5g of fat per serving
Low-fat	3g of fat or less per serving
Reduced fat	At least 25 percent less fat per serving than a comparable food
Sodium-free	Less than 5mg of sodium per serving
Low in sodium	140mg of sodium or less per serving
Reduced sodium	At least 25 percent less sodium per serving than a comparable food
Sugar-free	Less than 0.5g of sugar per serving
Reduced sugar	At least 25 percent less sugar per serving than a comparable food
High, Rich In, or Excellent Source of	Contains 20 percent or more of the daily value (DV) of that particular nutrient
Good Source, Contains, or Provides	Contains 10 to 19 percent of the daily value (DV) of that particular nutrient
More, Fortified, Enriched, Added, Extra, or Plus	Contains at least 10 percent more of the daily value (DV) of a particular nutrient than a comparable food
Lean	Contain less than 10g total fat, 4.5g or less saturated fat, and less than 95mg cholesterol per serving (on seafood or meat products)
Extra lean	Contains less than 5g total fat, less than 2g saturated fat, and less than 95mg cholesterol per serving (on seafood or meat products)

Identifying healthy protein choices

While you might expect to head to the meat department for your protein needs, you'll find potential choices in almost every section of the grocery store. Understanding this fact can be helpful if you're on a budget. Meat and seafood tend to be pricier than some plant-based options, like dry beans.

Figure 8-1 is a list of protein foods in different sections of the grocery store. The foods are specifically *not* identified as good foods or healthy foods simply because what is a good food for one person's diet might not be a good food for another person's diet. But it is always helpful to consider a wide range of options.

Also, some of these foods contain more protein than others. For example, cottage cheese provides much more protein per serving than asparagus. But asparagus provides more protein than many other fruit and veggie options in the produce section. It is included in the list so that people who want to get protein from veggies and other plant-based foods know what their options are in the produce section. And remember, almost all foods contain more than one macronutrient. So, you might see some foods on multiple lists.

Scan this list and choose the options that you want to add to your own grocery list. Or copy the entire list and take it with you when you go to the market.

Identifying healthy carbohydrate choices

There is no shortage of carbohydrate foods in any supermarket, but many of them contain high amounts of added sugar, which may not align with your healthy eating plan. Carbohydrate foods that will help you reach the nutritional recommendations provided by the USDA include grains, especially whole grains, fruits, vegetables, and other foods with fiber.

Figure 8-2 provides a list of carbohydrates that you might want to consider adding to your cart at the market. This is not a comprehensive list of every carb choice at the store, but these foods provide a range of nutrients while also helping you to reach your carb targets.

Identifying healthy fat choices

Many of the protein and carbohydrate foods that you buy will also contain fat. For example, red meats contain fat, primarily saturated fat. The American Heart Association suggests that we limit our intake of saturated fat to reduce the risk of heart disease. So, you may also want to consider fatty fish like salmon and tuna. Both varieties of fish contain omega-3 fatty acids, which are linked to health benefits rather than health risks.

Meat Department

☐ Beef (ground beef, steaks)
☐ Chicken (whole chicken or chicken parts)
☐ Duck
☐ Game meats (bear, bison, elk, etc.)
☐ Lamb
☐ Pork
☐ Sliced meats (chicken, turkey, ham)
☐ Turkey

Seafood Department

☐ Clams
☐ Crab
☐ Cod
☐ Flounder
☐ Lobster
☐ Mussels
☐ Octopus
☐ Oysters
☐ Salmon
☐ Scallops
☐ Seafood burgers or sausage
☐ Shrimp or other shellfish
☐ Squid
☐ Tilapia
☐ Trout (and other finfish)
☐ Tuna

Refrigerated Section

☐ Cottage cheese
☐ Eggs
☐ Egg whites
☐ Greek yogurt
☐ Hummus
☐ Milk
☐ Milk alternatives (soy, almond, oat, etc.)
☐ Pre-packaged protein smoothies
☐ Tempeh
☐ Tofu
☐ Yogurt

Produce and Bulk Food

☐ Asparagus
☐ Collard greens
☐ Broccoli
☐ Brussels sprouts
☐ Brown rice
☐ Dry beans
☐ Kale
☐ Lentils
☐ Nuts (almonds, walnuts, pistachios, etc.)
☐ Quinoa
☐ Seeds (chia, flax, pumpkin, etc.)
☐ Spinach

Canned and Dry Goods

☐ Canned beans (black beans, kidney beans, chick peas, split peas, etc.)
☐ Canned (or pouch) chicken
☐ Canned (or pouch) tuna
☐ Canned (or pouch) salmon
☐ Dried beans
☐ High-protein breakfast cereals
☐ Nutritional yeast
☐ Other canned fish (sardines, herring, etc.)
☐ Peanut butter and other nut butters
☐ Powdered egg whites
☐ Protein bars
☐ Sprouted grain bread
☐ Tahini
☐ Whole-wheat or chickpea pasta
☐ Wild rice

Frozen Foods

☐ Edamame
☐ High-protein meals
☐ High-protein treats
☐ Lima beans
☐ Meats and poultry
☐ Peas
☐ Plant-based sausage
☐ Soy- or plant-based meat alternatives
☐ Spinach

FIGURE 8-1: Protein foods by grocery store section.

Canned and Dry Goods	Produce and Bulk Food
☐ Applesauce	☐ Apples
☐ Bagels	☐ Asparagus
☐ Beans (including baked beans)	☐ Bananas
☐ Biscuits	☐ Barley
☐ Bread (including whole-grain bread)	☐ Beets
☐ Canned fruit	☐ Berries
☐ Cereal	☐ Bulk grains (millet, farro, quinoa, etc.)
☐ Cornbread	☐ Cabbage or slaw mix
☐ Crackers (including whole-grain crackers)	☐ Carrots
☐ Dried fruit	☐ Cauliflower
☐ English muffins	☐ Cherries
☐ Hot cereal (oats, oatmeal, grits)	☐ Citrus fruit
☐ Muffins or muffin mixes	☐ Corn
☐ Naan	☐ Couscous
☐ Pancake or waffle mixes	☐ Granola
☐ Pasta (including whole-grain pasta)	☐ Grapes
☐ Pita bread	☐ Leafy greens (spinach, kale, mustard greens, etc.)
☐ Polenta	☐ Lentils
☐ Popcorn	☐ Mushrooms
☐ Pretzels and snack foods	☐ Onions
☐ Raisins	☐ Peaches
☐ Rice (including wild and brown rice)	☐ Peppers
☐ Rice cakes	☐ Plums
☐ Tortillas (corn or flour)	☐ Squash
	☐ Tomatoes
	☐ Zucchini

Refrigerated Section	Frozen Foods
☐ Fresh pasta	☐ Berries
☐ Fruit juice	☐ Cauliflower rice
☐ Greek yogurt	☐ Corn
☐ Hummus	☐ Dough (pizza, pie, pastry)
☐ Milk	☐ Falafel
☐ Milk alternatives (soy, almond, oat, etc.)	☐ Fruit treats and other frozen desserts
☐ Pre-packaged smoothies	☐ Potatoes
☐ Tortillas	☐ Veggies (mixed veggies, peas, carrots, etc.)
☐ Vegetable juices	
☐ Yogurt	

FIGURE 8-2:
Carbohydrate foods by grocery store section.

Since fat is found in so many protein and carb foods, you won't need to put a lot of effort into buying fat-specific foods, because you will probably meet your intake targets with those protein and carb items. But these are some sources of fat that you might want to consider as well when you shop:

» Avocado

» Avocado oil

» Cheese

- » Dark chocolate

- » Flaxseed and flaxseed oil

- » Full-fat dairy

- » Nut butter (like peanut butter and almond butter)

- » Nuts and seeds

- » Olives and olive tapenade

- » Olive oil and other plant-based oils

Not all fatty foods will align with your nutritional goals. For instance, full-fat dairy might work for people who choose a higher fat intake, but not for those who are trying to reduce overall fat or saturated fatty foods.

REMEMBER

Remember to read nutritional labels to decide if a particular food aligns with your overall health and wellness goals.

Practicing Food Safety

Since you'll be preparing, storing, and reheating meals at home, it's important to follow smart food safety guidelines. You don't want a case of food poisoning to derail your efforts to reach the nutritional goals you've set for yourself.

The goal of food safety standards is to protect you and your family from foodborne illnesses or injuries related to food preparation and consumption.

So, I'll go over the basic guidelines regarding the handling, storing, and reheating of food.

TIP

If you're interested in learning more about staying safe in the kitchen, the U.S. government has an entire website dedicated to food safety tips, recalls, and news. Visit foodsafety.gov to learn more.

Food preparation tips

Meal prep involves chopping and mixing foods in large quantities. Simple practices can ensure that your food stays free from bacteria while you prepare it.

To avoid food-related illnesses, experts suggest that you follow these four rules:

>> Wash your hands with soap for at least 20 seconds before and after handling food.

>> Keep raw meat, poultry, fish, and their juices away from other food to avoid cross-contamination.

>> After cutting raw meats, clean the cutting board, knife, and countertops with hot soapy water.

>> Marinate meat and poultry in a covered dish in the refrigerator (never out on the counter).

REMEMBER

Putting your cutting boards in the dishwasher after every use will help to keep them clean, but not all cutting boards are dishwasher safe. Hand-wash wood cutting boards, thin plastic boards, and any other cutting board that doesn't specifically state that it is dishwasher safe.

Regardless of how you clean the cutting boards, you should also sanitize them occasionally. To sanitize your cutting boards, mix one tablespoon of unscented, liquid chlorine bleach in a gallon of water and use the solution to wipe down the boards. The Academy of Nutrition and Dietetics also suggests that you throw away any old cutting boards that have cracks, crevices, or excessive knife scars as bacteria can hide in those spaces.

REMEMBER

When cooking meat, poultry, and seafood, always use a meat thermometer and make sure that the food is cooked to the appropriate temperature provided in the recipe.

Food storage tips

After your meals are prepared, most of them will need to be refrigerated or frozen soon after.

REMEMBER

Always refrigerate or freeze perishable foods within two hours of cooking. If the temperature outside is greater than 90 degrees, refrigerate the food within one hour.

Your refrigerator should maintain a temperature of 40 degrees or below, and the freezer should maintain a temperature of at least 0 degrees. Also, it is a good idea to divide large food dishes into smaller, shallow containers for quicker cooling. For this reason and for convenience, it's a good idea to use single-serve containers for your prepped meals.

Keep in mind that frozen foods remain safe indefinitely, according to the USDA, although food quality can start to deteriorate after 1-2 months (depending on the type of food).

When your food is refrigerated, you need to be sure that the food is consumed within the recommended time frame. The amount of time varies for different foods, but here are some recommendations for popular foods.

>> Casseroles: 3 to 4 days

>> Cooked chicken breast: 3 to 4 days

>> Cooked ground meat or poultry: 3 to 4 days

>> Egg dishes: 3 to 4 days

>> Grains (rice, quinoa, oats): 4 to 6 days

>> Hard-boiled eggs: One week

>> Roasted vegetables: 3 to 7 days

>> Seafood and shellfish: 3 to 4 days

>> Sliced deli meats: 3 to 5 days

Tips for reheating food

The microwave oven is most commonly used for reheating meals that have been prepped in advance. It's so convenient to pull your meal out of the refrigerator and have it hot and ready to eat in just a few minutes. But not all microwave ovens work the same. While they all use the same technology to heat food, the wattage of the ovens can vary.

Microwave ovens may have wattage as low as 300 to 500 watts or as high as 1,000 watts or more. When cooking or reheating food, use less time for high-wattage ovens and more time for lower-wattage ovens.

For any wattage oven, use these guidelines provided by the USDA:

>> Use a microwave-safe container and cover food with a lid or with plastic wrap for even cooking. Be sure to vent the lid to allow steam to escape.

>> To ensure uniform cooking, arrange your food items evenly in the dish. You may need to add some liquid to dishes that include foods like rice or pasta.

>> Halfway through the cooking process, stir or rotate your food to help it cook more evenly. Foods should be stirred even if you have a rotating plate in your microwave oven.

>> Heat foods until steaming hot.

>> When cooking is complete, allow a resting time of 3 minutes or more.

>> Use a food thermometer to make sure your meal has reached a temperature of 165 degrees.

Food continues to cook after it has been removed from the oven. So, if you're testing the temperature of your meal, wait until the resting time is complete.

With some experimentation, you'll learn exactly how long it takes to reheat food in your oven. And you'll learn which foods work best for microwave reheating.

TIP

In general, foods that reheat well in the microwave include casseroles, soups, stews, egg dishes, steamed vegetables, rice, pasta, chili, many baked goods, oats, and other foods with higher moisture content.

If you don't own a microwave or if you prefer not to use one, you can also use your standard oven, a toaster oven, or the cooktop to reheat prepped meals. Reheating food on the stove or in the oven gives you more control over the temperature, and foods are more likely to cook evenly, but it takes longer.

For stovetop reheating, plan to cook a single prepped meal for about 5 minutes in a covered saucepan with a lid (the lid traps steam, which helps to cook the food more quickly). Be sure to stir every minute or so.

When reheating foods in the oven or toaster oven, you'll have to take into account preheating time (which will be longer in a standard oven). To reheat a single meal in the toaster oven, plan for 2 to 4 minutes. A standard oven is likely to take 5 to 10 minutes (depending on your oven's efficiency). Stirring halfway through is usually not necessary.

If you have leftovers after reheating and enjoying your prepped meal, it is safe to put them back in the refrigerator for 3 to 4 days, according to the USDA. But food quality diminishes with each reheating.

TIP

When prepping meals, try to put only a single portion in each meal container.

Fine-tuning Your Macro Meal Timing

When you eat can have an effect on whether or not you reach your macro diet goals. In fact, if you look at many macro diet social media sites, you'll see influencers discuss meal timing almost as often as they discuss macro targets and other components of the diet.

In general, it is smart to eat when you're hungry. Sounds simple, right? If you can listen to your body's cues, you would eat when you feel hungry and stop eating when you feel full and satisfied. Unfortunately, however, we are not always prepared when hunger hits.

TIP

Nutrient timing is a key concern, especially for athletes. The term "nutrient timing" refers to the methodical planning of food (or supplement) intake to maximize recovery, muscle tissue repair, and improved mood after high-volume or intense exercise. Nutrient timing may also be important for people who are trying to lose weight or who get uncomfortable hunger pangs throughout the day.

The International Society of Sports Nutrition (ISSN) and other researchers have investigated different strategies to provide guidelines about the best time to consume macronutrients, especially protein and carbs. You can implement these guidelines if you'd like. But dietary timing shouldn't take precedence over diet quality.

REMEMBER

Eating a balanced diet should be a higher priority than the perfect timing of your meals — even for athletes. Nutrient timing is part of the fine-tuning process that *can* be — but doesn't necessarily *need* to be — a component of your comprehensive macro diet plan.

So, take the following guidelines into account and use them as much as you'd like in your schedule. But don't worry if your timing isn't perfect. What matters more is the quality of your overall diet.

Timing your protein intake

For general health and wellness, including at least some protein in all of your meals and snacks is a smart approach. Then your body gets important amino acids to build and repair tissue regularly throughout the day.

REMEMBER

Nutrition experts often advise that you consume three meals per day with a couple of snacks in between meals. That way, you'll be getting some protein every three to four hours.

In a published paper on nutrient timing, the International Society of Sports Nutrition (ISSN) also suggests that people who exercise for general fitness should meet their overall protein needs by consuming protein approximately every three hours during the day.

Keep in mind, however, that these are general guidelines. Some people may prefer fewer meals, and some might need to eat more often. It is fine to experiment with a schedule to learn your optimal eating frequency for general wellness.

If your goal is weight loss, you may want to take your schedule and your hunger levels into consideration when you fine-tune your protein intake schedule.

REMEMBER

Some studies have suggested that consuming protein can help you to manage hunger hormones throughout the day. Research has even linked a higher-protein breakfast with better weight-loss outcomes.

If you are using the macro diet to reach and maintain a healthy weight (and weight loss is part of that goal), then you may want to think about your day and identify the times when you are most likely to get hungry. Do you start to get cravings in the late morning (as many of us do!) or do your hunger pangs hit later in the afternoon?

TIP

If you can boost your protein intake an hour or so before cravings typically hit, then you may be able to ward off the discomfort that comes from hunger.

Having a quick protein snack or a meal with protein may help prevent a visit to the office vending machine or a detour to the drive-thru window, when your stomach starts to growl and you need food quickly. Remember, protein takes longer to digest, so you are more likely to feel full and satisfied longer after a protein-rich meal or snack.

If your macro diet goals are athletic, particularly if you want to build muscle mass, then timing your protein intake may be of particular importance. Specifically, sports nutrition experts suggest consuming protein shortly after your workout.

REMEMBER

Various experts have suggested that you consume high-quality protein within two hours after exercise. To maximize your muscle-building potential, this feeding should include 20 to 40 grams of total protein with about 10 grams of essential amino acids.

To accomplish this nutrition goal, many strength-trained athletes consume a protein smoothie after their workout. Chapter 14 includes recipes for smoothies that you can try.

In addition to getting protein throughout the day and directly after exercise, strength-trained athletes may also benefit from getting a dose before bedtime.

TIP

The ISSN suggests consuming about 30 to 40 grams of casein protein at night to boost metabolism and improve muscle protein synthesis (building and repairing muscle tissue) throughout the night.

Timing your intake of carbs

When considering the timing of your carbohydrate intake, it is helpful to remember that carbs provide energy. So, you want to consume carbohydrates when you know you'll need to get — and stay — energized, such as during a workout.

Endurance athletes, like runners or cyclists, need to be especially careful about carbohydrate intake before exercise. These athletes need energy for extended bouts of activity, sometimes lasting several hours. But strength-trained athletes can also benefit from adding some carbs to their pre-workout or post-workout snack. And anyone who exercises can use these guidelines to be sure they are properly fueled for activity.

TIP

For a workout lasting less than an hour, a light snack consisting of mostly carbohydrates with a little bit of protein 30 minutes before exercise will help you maintain your energy.

For example, you might have a banana with a tablespoon of peanut butter. Another popular pre-workout carb/protein snack is a glass of chocolate milk.

If you participate in longer workouts lasting 90 minutes or more, experts generally advise consuming carbohydrates during the workout. Experts often suggest getting about 30 to 60 grams of carbs per hour or even up to 90 grams of carbs per hour for very long sessions.

TIP

To avoid stomach problems and for reasons of convenience, many exercisers and athletes turn to supplements (in liquid or gel form) to meet these needs.

On days when you don't work out (or for people who don't exercise), timing your carb intake doesn't need to be complicated. You'll want to consume carbs at every meal just to be sure that you're meeting your daily needs with a steady intake. Aside from that, you can take the *type* of carbs into consideration when planning your meals.

Choose fiber-rich carbohydrates when you need longer-duration sustainable energy. Foods like oatmeal, whole-wheat bread, or legumes will give you longer-lasting energy. If you need a quick burst of energy, choose quick energy sources, like a bagel or fresh fruit (oranges, grapes, or berries).

Timing your intake of fat

Unless you are on a diet that prioritizes fat (like the ketogenic diet), you probably don't need to worry about timing your fat intake. For most of us, we get plenty of fat in the normal preparation and consumption of food.

For instance, you might use oil to cook fish or meat at dinner time. You might add avocado or butter to your toast in the morning, or yogurt in the afternoon, and unless you choose the fat-free variety, you'll get a few grams of fat in those foods.

Since fat provides twice as many calories per gram as carbohydrates and protein, you'll meet your recommended intake with far less food volume. Simply put, a little goes a long way!

REMEMBER

Whatever timing pattern you choose for protein, for carbs, and for fat, just remember to make your plan sustainable. In the end, diet quality is your top priority, and consistency matters as well. So, if timing your intake of macros seems overwhelming, don't worry about it for now.

First, focus on enjoying a range of nutritious foods and meeting your macro targets. If meal prep is going to be a part of your regular macro diet routine, then your next priority can be getting your meal prep routine dialed in. After you feel like a macro diet pro, then revisit the idea of timing. You'll get the most out of this eating plan when you take it one step at a time.

Chapter 9

Monitoring Your Progress and Making Changes

Y ou'll set a goal for yourself at the beginning of your macro diet journey. You may even set several goals for yourself. But those goals are not set in stone, nor are the targets you calculate for yourself when coming up with your macro numbers. You can — and should — make adjustments from time to time. This reevaluation process ensures that your goals are realistic and attainable and will help to keep you on track.

In this chapter, I walk you through the reevaluation process. I show you how and when to revisit your goals and targets and the type of adjustments you can make based on your needs. I also give you some ideas to consider for your future plan. Most people don't follow the macro diet forever. So, this chapter helps you turn your macro diet into a sustainable long-term program so that you maintain the nutritional gains you worked so hard to achieve.

Knowing When You Should Assess

Everyone's diet journey is unique. So, there is no single answer for when to start reevaluating your program. But you'll definitely want to modify your targets if you notice any red flags, like a negative relationship with food or poor body image. Even if things seem to be going well, you should check in and reassess often, and you can rely on your SMART goals (Chapter 4) to help you determine the right time.

Looking out for red flags

REMEMBER

Your diet might be "working" in that you're able to stick to it and you're making steady progress to reach your designated goal. But sometimes, other issues arise that are problematic and warrant your attention. If being on the macro diet negatively changes your relationship with food, induces stress, or causes you to make lifestyle changes that don't serve your best interests, then it's *not* working.

If you have concerns, ask yourself these questions about your experience with the macro eating plan. If you're unsure about how the diet affects your mental well-being, read Chapter 4.

» **Do I enjoy the foods and meals on the diet?** Do I look forward to mealtime? Do I feel satiated after eating? Am I getting enough food variety to stay interested in the meal plan? Food satisfaction and enjoyment are crucial for long-term adherence. If you answered no to any of these questions, you may need to tweak your diet to include foods that you enjoy and that make you feel good.

» **Are any areas of my life taking a backburner to my diet?** Does my eating plan interfere with my daily routine, work schedule, or social activities? It's fine to prioritize good nutrition, but you shouldn't feel like you're making significant life sacrifices to eat a specific way. If you feel like a slave to your eating plan, it's not sustainable.

» **Am I experiencing any negative mental or physical side effects as a result of being on the macro diet?** How do I feel if I don't hit my targets on a given day? You might want to monitor your self-talk and thoughts as they relate to food. If you find yourself feeling "bad" about certain food choices, the eating plan might not be sustainable. There are better ways to foster good nutrition.

» **How does the diet make me feel emotionally?** Has the diet affected my body image or my relationship with food? Eating a nutritious diet should help you to feel strong and empowered and promote a healthy relationship with food. Your diet is unhealthy when it negatively changes your self-image or makes you feel bad about eating.

If you're concerned about any of these red flags, seek the help of a professional. Nutrition and behavioral health specialists can help you to develop an eating plan that meets your goals and allows you to feel good about your food choices and your body image.

Timing your check-ins

If you set a SMART goal, you may have a built-in assessment schedule already in mind. In Chapter 5, I explain that SMART goals are specific, measurable, attainable, relevant, and time-bound. The last element, "time-bound," can help indicate when it's time to check in. For instance, if you set a goal to lose 10 pounds in three months, you will already have a check-in scheduled at the three-month mark.

Usually, however, you'll want to check in before that — especially when you're first starting out. But you also need to give yourself time to adapt to your new program. The beginning of the macro diet will be the most challenging. At this stage, you're learning new skills and making (potentially) major changes to the way you fuel your body. It takes time for your brain and your body to adjust.

Give yourself at least a month to start the macro diet before checking in or making significant changes. You may see some benefits within the first week or so — such as changes to your energy level or to your hunger levels throughout the day. But it will take much longer to see changes in weight, athletic performance, or body composition.

If you're able to be consistent on the plan for a month or so, then you can re-assess at that point. But if not, give it a little bit more time. You may need to try a different tracking method or a new meal planning schedule to fine-tune your process. But, if you can't be consistent on the program after about six weeks, this may indicate that your goals aren't attainable. A check-in at that point is warranted.

After you make initial adjustments to your plan, continue to check in every few months until you reach your goal. But you should also be mindful of changes in your life that might suggest a change or reevaluation of your plan. These changes might include:

>> A change in your exercise/physical activity level

>> Changes to your daily routine that might affect your food intake

>> A change in your health status

>> Unintentional changes to your weight

Any change that might affect your ability to stick to your plan or your body's energy needs should warrant a reassessment of your diet. Changes to your health status or unintended weight changes may also warrant a visit to your healthcare provider. You may find that no changes need to be made, but having the confidence of knowing that might help you stay on track for the long term.

Checking Your Progress

You can determine if your diet is working in several ways. The goal you set for yourself can be your primary indicator. For instance, if you set a goal to lose 10 pounds in three months and you're already at your goal weight at week 10, then you can assume that your program is on track. But it usually isn't that simple.

Reaching (or not reaching) your primary goal is the simplest way to indicate whether or not the macro diet is successful. But you should stay open to other changes that might be happening as well. You may experience unexpected outcomes that can help to indicate that the program is working for you in unanticipated ways.

For instance, the scale isn't always the best indicator of whether or not your diet is successful. You can use body composition measurements, your clothing fit, athletic assessments, or even just noticing how you feel each day to determine if you're on track. In this section, I explain different ways to help you determine if you should change your diet or stick with your program as is.

Weight: The traditional method

For years, dieters who were trying to lose weight have used a bathroom scale to determine if they were successful on their program. In fact, some research studies have even shown that daily weigh-ins can improve weight loss outcomes. But there are pros and cons to using this tried-and-true tactic.

On the upside, the scale is an inexpensive and simple way to see if you've lost weight. While you can pay hundreds of dollars or more for a scale, a simple and accurate bathroom scale can be purchased for $30 or less. It doesn't take up a lot of room in your home and is easy to use. Many digital scales even store your data so that you can track changes over time on a website or smartphone app.

But the number you see on the scale doesn't always tell the full story. A significant increase or decrease in your weight doesn't necessarily mean that you've lost or gained fat. If you weigh yourself on a different scale, for instance, you may see a different number simply because the equipment is different. For this reason, you should always try to weigh yourself on the same scale at the same time of day.

Another issue is frequency. If you weigh yourself too often, you may notice normal fluctuations that don't necessarily indicate fat loss. Keep in mind that there is no need to weigh yourself every day. Weekly (or even biweekly) weigh-ins are perfectly fine and may be more accurate.

REMEMBER

Many factors can affect your weight from day to day. In fact, weight fluctuations of five pounds or even more are common and should be expected.

Usually, weight fluctuations throughout the day are due to water weight changes. These factors can cause weight increases or decreases that are not related to fat loss:

>> Dehydration from alcohol intake

>> Dehydration from exercise

>> Water retention from hormonal shifts

>> Water retention from sodium intake

>> Weight fluctuations from medications

You wouldn't want to throw your program out the window because of temporary changes in your water weight.

REMEMBER

Your diet might be working, and you might be losing weight in a healthy way, but the scale may not show success because of simple water weight changes or technical issues.

Another important downside to using a scale is that it can have negative psychological outcomes. Several studies have tied self-weighing to poor self-esteem and negative body image in some people, especially women and younger individuals. While this isn't everyone's experience, you should be aware that self-weighing can sometimes do more harm than good.

WARNING

For some people, the experience of getting on the scale is emotionally harmful, leading to feelings of frustration, disappointment, and distress. If you have *any* reservations about using the scale, then don't use it! There's absolutely nothing wrong with ditching the scale for good.

Many other (more accurate) ways exist to determine if your macro diet is working. One of those methods is measuring body composition.

Body composition: Muscle, fat, and all that

Body composition is a term that describes the ratio of fat mass to lean mass (muscle and bone) on your body. When body composition is measured, you get a body fat percentage as the result of whatever testing method you use.

Body composition takes into account more than just total body weight, so it's often a better indicator of changes in body fat than using a simple scale.

Like the scale, using body composition measurements has pros and cons. For some people, the tests are highly relevant. For instance, if you set a goal to build muscle mass and reduce body fat, these tests (when measured and compared over time) can tell you how much lean mass (muscle) you gained and how much fat mass you lost. A basic scale can't do that. These tests can also be useful for people who have set a weight loss goal.

It's not uncommon for people to gain muscle but lose fat when they pair a macro diet with an exercise program. On a basic scale, this may show up as weight gain (or no weight change at all) and can lead to feelings of failure or frustration. A body composition test, however, can indicate fat loss and muscle mass gains, leading to feelings of improved confidence and success.

But for some people, the test will be less relevant. For instance, if you set a more generalized goal to improve your health (such as boosting daily energy levels or feeling better throughout the day), a body composition measurement can't necessarily reveal whether you've met your goal.

You can use several different methods to get your body fat percentage. The options vary in price, availability, and accuracy. Following are some of the more popular methods available.

>> **BodPod:** This large egg-shaped device measures body fat using air displacement technology. It can also estimate metabolic rates. To do the test, you sit inside the enclosed device for about 10 minutes while measurements are taken. The test is non-invasive and completely comfortable for most people. People who do not like being in small, enclosed spaces may not feel comfortable, but you can stop the test at any time. Test results are considered to be very accurate.

>> **Body fat calculator:** Plenty of online calculators estimate body fat percentage using your weight and various body measurements such as wrist, forearm, waist, or hip. The measurements needed are different for men and women. While this method is completely free and easy to use, it's not considered to be very accurate.

>> **Bioelectrical impedance (BIA):** Your home scale may measure body fat using BIA technology. Scales in gyms, clinics, and even your doctor's office may also use bioelectrical impedance to estimate body fat percentage. BIA devices send a harmless, pain-free electrical signal through your body to give you instantaneous results. While this method is convenient, certain factors, such as hydration level, can influence the accuracy of the result.

>> **DeXA scanning:** This test involves whole-body scanning and is usually only available in clinical settings. But it's quickly becoming the gold standard for measuring body fat. The test is performed by medical technicians who are highly trained in various radiological procedures. While the test is highly accurate, it's often costly and may not be available outside of your medical provider's office.

>> **Hydrostatic weighing:** During this test, you'll immerse yourself in water. Based on the amount of water you displace, technicians are able to estimate your body fat percentage. For many years, this test was considered the gold standard for measuring body fat, but many people are not comfortable being fully immersed in water or holding their breath. In addition, this test can be costly and is often only available in lab settings.

>> **Skin caliper measurements:** If you go to a gym or health club, trainers often use skin calipers to measure body fat (although BIA scales and devices have become more common in recent years). By measuring skin folds in various body spots (the locations are different for men and women), your trainer can estimate your total body fat percentage. This method is only as accurate as the person who performs the test. If the trainer is highly skilled, then you will probably get an accurate result. But if the skin fold measurements are not taken properly, then you can get a faulty result.

TIP

Whatever method you choose to measure body composition, you should stick with that method as you measure your progress over time to ensure accuracy. For instance, if you went to your local health club and had a trainer do skin caliper measurements, then your follow-up measurements should be done with those same calipers, and the same trainer should conduct the test. That way, you minimize the chances that the testing method (or user error) plays a role in any change you see in your body fat.

Clothing fit: A little loose, a little tight, or just right

If you've set a weight-loss goal for your macro diet journey and you don't want to get on the scale or pay for body composition tests, you have a simple and cost-free method of measuring your progress: your clothing fit.

TIP

Simply paying attention to how your clothes fit is the easiest way to know if you're on track for reaching your weight loss goals on the macro diet. You're gonna get dressed in the morning anyway!

If you're on the path to losing weight, you can take an extra minute or two to see how loose your waistband feels, how snug your jeans feel through the hips, how your tank top feels on your chest, or how well the zipper goes up on your dress. You might even snap a quick smartphone pic and revisit the image in a week or two to compare the looks. Small improvements might give you an extra boost of energy and encouragement. But as you might imagine, this method has some downsides, too.

REMEMBER

Clothing fit does not take into account daily fluctuations in your size due to water weight changes. Clothing fit also can't distinguish between changes in body size due to muscle gains or fat loss — which can happen when you pair the macro diet with an exercise program.

Fitness trainers sometimes tell their clients to use clothing fit rather than the scale to indicate improvements in body composition. They make this suggestion because gaining muscle while losing fat can mean that your body gets heavier but slightly smaller and tighter — so your clothes would feel a bit more loosely. Even though your scale won't show the results of your hard work, it's easy to notice when you get dressed in the morning.

But it's very difficult to gain muscle while losing fat. So, there may be stages during your macro diet journey when you gain muscle without significant fat loss. As a result, your clothes might get a little tighter, even though you're on track and making improvements. All of these conflicting situations can make clothing fit a tricky method to use when measuring progress.

WEIGHING MUSCLE VERSUS FAT

Whether you're using the scale or clothing fit to measure progress on your macro diet journey, it's helpful to understand the difference between muscle and fat when it comes to body weight and body size.

Muscle is denser than fat. So, muscle weighs more but takes up less space on your body. If you were to gain one pound of muscle while losing one pound of fat, your body would be slightly smaller, even though there would be a slight increase on the scale. But we usually don't gain muscle and lose fat in equal proportions, so it's hard to know what's going on when there are changes to the way your clothes fit or when you see changes on the scale. This is one more reason why many exercisers choose body composition measurements over clothing fit or simple body fat scales for measuring progress.

Another problem with using clothing fit as a measurement of progress is that it puts the focus on your outward appearance.

REMEMBER

You might be feeling more energized and confident as a result of making healthy changes to your diet. It's important to give yourself credit for those accomplishments, regardless of how your clothes fit or what the scale says.

Performance: Jump a little higher, run a little faster

If you set an athletic goal for yourself and you're using the macro diet to support your training efforts, you may not care what the scale says or how your clothes fit. You want to know if your performance is improving.

Many athletes already have testing and measurement protocols in place to track their training. For instance, a trainer at your local gym might give you a treadmill test to evaluate your cardiovascular fitness. If you're a strength-trained athlete, your trainer might evaluate the maximum amount of weight you can lift in one repetition for various exercises.

To make sure that you get an accurate assessment of your training progress, be sure to test at the very beginning of your training journey. This provides a baseline that you can use to compare future test results.

Then when you reevaluate, be sure to use the same testing equipment, location, or methods so that you know you're comparing apples to apples.

Keep in mind that fitness tests don't necessarily give you confirmation that the *diet* is effective because the diet itself isn't evaluated. But if you're using the diet to support your athletic training, it can help confirm that the nutritional planning is working as expected.

But what if you set a more generalized goal? Perhaps you're not a hardcore runner or a serious weightlifter. Maybe you've set a goal to simply get in shape or improve your overall level of fitness and you're using the macro diet to work hand in hand with a new exercise program.

You can do several different tests on your own to measure various performance improvements. Consider using one of these methods to evaluate your training and diet progress.

One-mile walk test

This test is a variation of the *Rockport test*, a walking protocol often used by exercise physiologists to estimate VO2 max — the maximum volume of oxygen that your body can use during exercise. The higher the number, the better your heart and lungs work during exercise. This number generally improves as you get fitter.

TIP

The one-mile walk test is a simple variation of the Rockport test that physiologists often perform. It can be used to measure your progress if you're using the macro diet to support a program of aerobic or cardiovascular training.

To conduct the test, you simply measure how long it takes you to walk a mile. You can do this test on a track at your local high school or college, or conduct the test on a walking path where you know the start and end points for one mile. You can also use a fitness tracker or smartwatch to measure a one-mile distance.

You'll want to warm up for about five minutes before starting the test. Then walk as briskly as possible for one mile and record your time. If you do this test at the beginning of your diet and fitness journey, you can retest every month or so to evaluate your progress. You should see that you can walk just a little bit faster each time.

Push-up test

This test is similar to the walking test, but instead of measuring your walking time, you will count the number of push-ups you can do in one minute.

The results of a push-up test will give you an idea of improvements in your upper body strength and endurance. This would be a good test to use if you have paired your macro diet with a program of strength training.

To do the test, set a timer for one minute. You can also have a friend or family member operate the timer. Get into position to start your push-up either on the floor (in a full push-up position or with the knees on the floor) or near a wall (to do a standing push-up). Then complete as many push-ups in that position as you can in one minute.

TIP

Make sure that you complete every repetition in the same position as you started. For example, if you started in a full push-up position with the hands and toes on the floor, then every rep should be completed in that position. You should not put your knees down halfway through the minute.

Record the number of push-ups completed. Retest in a couple of months or so to see improvements in your training.

REMEMBER

Keep in mind that fitness tests don't specifically tell you if the diet is working because they don't test the diet specifically. But they can help you to determine if the diet is working together with your exercise program to improve your health.

If you don't see improvements, you may need to make adjustments to your fitness training plan. But you can also reevaluate your diet if you feel that you don't have the energy to complete regular workouts.

Lifestyle factors: Feeling better, doing more

You can track your progress on the macro diet, even if your goal is to improve your overall sense of well-being. When you start to track your macros and start to consume a balanced diet, you're likely to see general health changes. For many people, this is the primary reason that they start and maintain the macro diet — they simply want to feel better!

If your health goals are specific (for example, lower cholesterol levels or better blood pressure readings), you can work with your healthcare provider to get initial tests and follow-up tests completed. But if your health goals are more general, you can use a journal to track changes in things like energy, mood, and sleep to see if your diet is working.

Energy

When you're getting the right number of calories and especially carbohydrates, you're likely to feel a better sense of steady energy throughout the day.

TIP

Before you start the macro diet, you might want to jot down the times during the day when you're likely to feel tired. For instance, many people experience an energy dip late in the morning or around 3 or 4 in the afternoon. After a few weeks on the macro diet, take note of how you feel during those time slots.

A journal is a great way to track these changes. Hopefully, your diet has given you a little bit more pep. But if not, you can make adjustments to your diet or your meal timing to get the energy you need (I cover the type of changes you can make in "Making Adjustments").

Mood

Your diet can affect your mood. If you started the macro diet to feel better emotionally, you can monitor your progress by becoming mindful of your feelings throughout the day and tracking those feelings in your journal.

For instance, it's not uncommon for your mood to take a dip when you haven't eaten in a while. We've all been hangry from time to time. Even though "hangry" isn't a real medical term, scientific researchers have noted that people can become aggressive, distractable, and impulsive when they are very hungry and their blood sugar plummets.

TIP

Before you start the macro diet, jot down how often and how intensely you experience mood changes related to hunger. Then check in weekly with your journal after you start changing your diet. You're likely to notice that you feel steadier and calmer. This often happens when you consume balanced nutrients throughout the day.

When you start to consume a balanced meal plan, you're more likely to avoid the blood sugar fluctuations that can impact your mood. If you can consume protein, healthy-fats, and carbs (especially fiber-rich carbs) at each meal or snack, you're more likely to experience a feeling of fullness and satisfaction for longer after eating.

Sleep

No single diet is known to improve sleep, but if you consume a wide variety of foods on the macro diet, especially fruits and vegetables, you're more likely to get the vitamins and minerals you need to get a restful night's sleep.

TIP

Researchers have found that if you're deficient in certain nutrients, such as calcium, magnesium, and vitamins A, C, D, E, and K, you're more likely to have sleep problems.

If sleep was an issue for you before starting the macro diet, keep a sleep log to track how often you wake during the night or how long it takes you to fall asleep. If you have a fitness monitor, you might be able to use that as well. Many of them track sleep quality along with other fitness factors.

Then after you start the macro diet, see if you experience any changes. If you do, then you can use this measure to help keep you motivated to stick to your plan. But if you don't, then you may want to evaluate the timing of your meals (try not to eat a big meal too close to bedtime) and make sure you're getting enough foods that contain those vital vitamins and minerals.

Making Adjustments

If you have decided that your macro diet needs adjusting, there are some basic changes you might want to consider. Some simple tweaks can help you to improve your energy, reduce hunger throughout the day, or boost weight loss.

Changes to increase energy

It's fairly common for your energy to lag when following a restrictive diet. But the macro diet should not feel restrictive. So, if hunger is nagging you throughout the day, it's important to make changes. Your body is telling you that it needs more than the diet is currently providing.

Consider these adjustments:

REMEMBER

>> **Increase your carb intake.** Does your carbohydrate intake fall within the guidelines set by the USDA?

The nutrition experts and the USDA advise that you consume between 45 to 65 percent of your daily calories from carbohydrates. Some popular macro ratios fall below that. For instance, if you're using the 40/30/30 plan, you might not be getting the carbohydrates that you need.

Try increasing your carb intake by 5 to 10 percent, especially at the meals you consume before the windows of time when you tend to feel tired.

>> **Adjust your caffeine consumption.** How much coffee do you consume each day? Are you guzzling down caffeinated sodas in the afternoon? Caffeine can temporarily increase alertness, but it can also make you feel tired after the initial buzz wears off.

The U.S. Food and Drug Administration suggests that we get no more than 400 milligrams of caffeine per day. That's about four or five cups of coffee. If you're drinking more than that, dial it back gradually to see if your energy levels improve.

>> **Drink more water.** Dehydration can make you feel sluggish. If your diet is on track, it's possible that your fluid intake is too low. Different recommendations for proper hydration exist, and some organizations simply suggest that you use thirst as a guide.

TECHNICAL STUFF

The U.S. National Academies of Sciences, Engineering, and Medicine suggests that men should get about 15.5 cups of fluids per day and women should get about 11.5 cups of fluids per day.

Keep in mind that you can drink water or other non-caffeinated beverages to reach these levels, but you can also increase your intake of hydrating foods, like melon, grapes, cucumber, or lettuce.

>> **Check your sleep hygiene.** One of the most obvious reasons for daytime fatigue is lack of sleep or poor-quality sleep at night. Poor-quality sleep can also impact the food choices you make during the day.

>> **Start or adjust your exercise program.** If you don't currently exercise, now might be the time to start. A regular program of exercise has been shown time and time again in research studies to increase feelings of energy throughout the day.

Changes to reduce hunger

Making any change to your diet can affect daily hunger levels.

REMEMBER

On the macro diet, you shouldn't feel like you're starving yourself. Restrictive diets are simply not sustainable (or healthy). If you have constant cravings, consider these changes.

>> **Adjust your fat intake.** Are you eating enough fat? This macronutrient was maligned for years — especially where weight loss is concerned. But it turns out that healthy fat is an important component of any diet, including diets for losing weight. Try making small adjustments to your fat intake and then give it a week to see how you feel. Add some avocado to your eggs in the morning, add a slice of cheese to your sandwich, or try swapping out the skim milk for 2 percent or full-fat milk in your cereal.

>> **Fill up on fiber-rich foods.** Foods with fiber help you to feel full longer after eating. Choose whole grains over enriched and processed grains when possible. Opt for whole-grain bread, whole-wheat pasta, and brown rice instead of white. Need a snack? Popcorn is full of fiber! You can also choose higher-fiber fruits and vegetables such as berries, broccoli, or pears.

>> **Get a serving of protein at every meal.** Protein digests slowly and keeps feelings of hunger at bay longer than quickly digesting sugary foods. Make sure that each meal and snack provides a portion of this macro. Foods like hard-boiled eggs, peanut butter and wheat crackers, or a handful of nuts make great snacks that can help keep cravings at bay.

>> **Question your cravings.** Sometimes, we think we are hungry, but we are really feeling bored, stressed, anxious, or even thirsty. When hunger hits, take a minute to analyze the sensation. Where do you feel it? Would a quick work break make you feel better? Can you grab a glass of water?

In some cases, that feeling in the pit of your stomach really *is* hunger and should be honored. But you may find that an emotion, like boredom or stress, is at play.

Changes to boost weight loss

What happens when your diet is going well, you enjoy your meals, you don't feel hungry, the plan seems manageable, but you're not losing weight? The problem may simply be that you need more time.

It's also possible that your weight goal isn't realistic. Have you been at your goal weight before? Did you set your goal in response to unrealistic social media images or pressure from others? If you know that your goal weight is healthy and realistic, consider these changes to boost your results.

>> **Begin an exercise program.** If you haven't started to exercise, now might be the best time to start. In addition to burning calories, it can help you to build muscle and boost your confidence, both of which can contribute to a successful weight-loss program. Start by choosing activities that you enjoy. If you don't like the gym, then don't go. Try bike riding, take a dance class, enroll in karate, or start swimming.

There are countless ways to get more active. Start with short, easy sessions 15 to 20 minutes long, 2 to 3 times per week and increase when you feel ready.

TIP

>> **Increase activity.** In Chapter 6, I explain how non-exercise activity thermogenesis (NEAT) contributes to the total number of calories per day. NEAT is all of the movement you do throughout the day that isn't exercise. It includes activities like walking to your car in the parking lot, carrying groceries into your house, gardening, or housecleaning. If you're a very active individual, it can burn hundreds of calories each day. See if you can increase this daily movement to boost your metabolism. If you work at a desk, set a timer every hour for a 5-minute movement break or take the stairs instead of the elevator. These small changes can really add up at the end of the day.

>> **Reduce calories.** Cutting down on your caloric intake can be tricky because if you go too low it can backfire. But it might be helpful to see where you're now and see if you can reduce it by 100 calories or so to start with. This might be as simple as opting for a cup of black coffee instead of the sweetened latte.

WARNING

Try to make changes slowly. Making a drastic change or cutting back too much can lead to binge eating or other disordered eating patterns. If you're unsure of the number of calories you should consume, talk to your healthcare provider and get a referral to see a registered dietitian. Many times, it takes just one session to get the information you need.

Determining How Long You Should Stay on the Macro Diet

One of the most common questions that people ask about the macro diet is: How long should I stay on it? The answer is different for everyone because everyone's goals are different.

Someone who set a goal to lose 50 pounds will obviously need to be on the diet for a longer period of time than someone who wants to lose 10 pounds. Similarly, using the macro diet to support your training to run a 5K will take less time than using the diet to support marathon training.

But after you've met your goal, now what? Should you stay on the macro diet forever?

Some people stay on the diet indefinitely. If you enjoy the meal prep process, you're getting the nutrients you need to feel energized and healthy throughout the day, and you enjoy a wide variety of nutritious foods, there is no reason to make changes.

But if you want to change things up, there are ways to make adjustments so that you maintain whatever gains you achieved during the active diet phase. You can either set a new goal, shift into a maintenance phase (see "Go into a maintenance phase"), or do periodic macro check-ins as a long-term strategy.

Set a new goal

Some people are goal-driven by nature. These people tend to be highly focused and organized. They also tend to be proactive and motivated. They are often described as being "type-A" personalities.

If that description sounds familiar, then you may want to set a new goal after reaching your initial target.

TIP

If you're a person who likes to keep an eye on the prize, you'll be served well by going through the SMART goal process (visit Chapter 5) and setting your sights on a new target.

So, what kind of new goal should you set? You can either use your first goal as a foundation and set the bar a little higher, or you can try a new type of goal altogether.

For instance, maybe your initial goal was to get in shape to complete a 5K run. For your next goal, you might find a longer race to complete, like a 10K. You'll need more time to train for that event, but you already know the basic diet and exercise plan to support your training. So, you can transition seamlessly into your new plan.

But maybe you'd like to try something different. For instance, if your first goal was to lose weight and you've reached your target number, you might set a new goal to gain muscle with a strength-training plan. You can still use the macro diet to support your new goal, but you will want to adjust your macro numbers to make sure that you get the right amount of protein to support your new program.

If you choose to set a new goal, keep in mind that it's okay (and often recommended) that you take some time off between reaching your old goal and setting a new one. Even just a week or two of more relaxed eating can help you to recharge so that you feel inspired and invigorated when you take on your new challenge.

This might mean that you eat whatever you want without counting every gram of protein, fat, and carbohydrate for a week or two. It might also mean that you focus on fun, easy workouts that you enjoy. Choose some way to reward yourself for the goal you just accomplished before tackling a new one.

Go into a maintenance phase

If you don't consider yourself to be type-A and you don't need a specific goal in mind to keep you inspired, you may want to ease into a maintenance phase after you reach your initial macro diet goal.

REMEMBER

A *maintenance phase* is a variation of the diet phase where you adjust your macronutrient and calorie targets to make them sustainable for the long term without undoing any progress that you made when you reached your initial goal.

The maintenance phase takes some trial and error, so you should expect to give yourself a few weeks to find out how much to adjust your calorie and macro numbers. You want to be sure to make small adjustments and make them gradually.

For instance, let's say that your initial macro diet goal was to lose 20 pounds. To reach your target, you consumed 1,500 calories per day with a macro balance of 50g of carbohydrates per day, 30g of protein per day, and 20g of fat per day. Now that you've reached your goal, you'd like to increase your fat intake slightly to enjoy some of the foods that you gave up during the weight loss phase.

Try increasing your calorie target by 100 calories per week. If you want to allocate those calories to your fat intake, you could consume about 11 more grams of fat per day (11 grams × 9 calories per gram = 99 calories). That would bring your fat intake to about 25 percent of your total calories — still within the nutritional recommendations established by the USDA.

You can give this plan a week or two and see if it affects your weight. If you're happy with the results, you can stick with your new plan or try adding another 100 calories if you feel like you'd like to eat a bit more. You can continue adding calories until you see your weight increase.

REMEMBER

Keep in mind that the number you calculated for your total daily calorie intake may have changed since you lost weight. Metabolism slows as you lose weight. If you lost a significant amount of weight, you may need to get your metabolism retested or reconfigure the number to take your new body size into account.

Track macros periodically

The last option for your long-term macro plan is to do occasional and intermittent tracking. That is, you stop tracking your macros every day. But you check in every once in a while to make sure you still consume a diet that supports good health and wellness. This is often a smart maintenance approach for people who set general wellness goals for themselves when they started the macro diet.

If you used the macro diet to learn how to eat a nutritionally balanced diet to support good health and you feel that you reached that goal, you don't have to continue to track your macros on a daily basis. Your maintenance phase can include one-week check-ins every few months to make sure you're still on the right track.

During each week-long assessment, you can track the nutrients you consume just like you did during the diet phase. You can use the same apps or tools that you used previously. Visit Chapter 7 to learn more about the apps and tools you can use for tracking.

During that week, you'll also want to be mindful of your overall sense of health and wellness. Are you still enjoying steady energy levels throughout the day? Do you have the fuel you need to support your workouts? Do you still enjoy your meals and feel satisfied after eating?

If the answers to these questions are yes, then give yourself another few months before checking in again. You can continue this pattern until you see a need to set a new goal. For instance, if your weight changes and you want to get it back on track, you can go back into an active macro diet phase. Or perhaps you want to take on a new athletic challenge, and you want to adjust your nutrient intake to support your training.

If, during your check-in period, you find that your macros have changed significantly from your original targets and your sense of wellness has dipped, then you might want to go back on the macro diet for a month or two to reestablish good nutritional habits and help you to get your balanced diet back on track.

Chapter **10**

Creating Your Daily Menus

Y ou might be wondering what a typical day of eating looks like on the macro diet. The great thing about this flexible plan is that you can choose the foods you want to enjoy. So, you can build a daily menu around foods you love.

There is no "right" food or "wrong" food on the macro diet. Your daily meal plan will probably look very different from someone else's plan. And that's okay! Your food preferences are unique, as are your goals and daily macro targets. These are the factors that will help you create the best meal plan for you.

Even though your meal plan will be unique, it can be helpful to see how meal plans with different calorie counts and macro targets might look. When you see how others set up their meals, it can help you to develop a sustainable plan for yourself.

In this chapter, I explain the different methods you might use to put together a daily meal plan for yourself. This chapter provides sample meal plans for different targets so that you can see how meals and snacks might be planned for different types of macro trackers. These are not recommended plans, just ideas that might work for different types of people.

As you scan through the sample plans, keep in mind that the meal and snack suggestions leave plenty of room for variation. That way, if you choose to use one of the meal suggestions or a full day's menu, you can tailor each meal to your own taste preferences.

Creating Your Own Meal Plan

You can take your macro targets and turn them into a meal plan for yourself in three different ways. You can use apps for part or all of the process. But some of them require a subscription or other fees. So, an alternate method is to do it yourself.

Do-it-yourself method

Many people who follow the macro diet, do so without the help of a tech tool. The DIY method is fairly straightforward. You simply use basic math to figure out how many macro grams and calories to allocate to each meal or snack. And since most people follow a similar eating schedule from day to day, you really only need to run the numbers once.

Follow these three simple steps.

1. If you have a calorie target, divide it by four. Then divide each of your daily macro targets by four. This will give you nutritional targets for three daily meals and two snacks. For instance, if your total daily calorie goal is 2,000 calories, then you'll consume 500 calories at each meal and have 500 calories to "spend" on snacks.

2. Divide your snack allotment by the number of snacks you plan to consume for the day. For example, if you want to have two snacks, divide 500 by 2. So, each snack should provide about 250 calories. Also follow this process for your macro targets.

3. Now use your targets to build a meal plan around foods that you enjoy. Start by choosing the foods you enjoy most and then adjust portion sizes as needed and add foods if necessary so that you reach your calorie and macro goals.

You can adjust this process according to the number of meals and/or snacks that you prefer. For example, some people are not snackers. So, they would divide their daily totals by 3 instead of 4 to account for three meals with no snacks.

You might also find that you prefer to have some meals that are smaller or larger than others. Simply adjust the numbers to your liking. In the preceding example, if you prefer to consume most of your calories earlier in day, you might consume 600 calories at breakfast, 600 at lunch, and 300 at dinner (keeping the snack allotment the same).

DIY + tracking app method

If you use the DIY method to figure out your targets for each meal and snack, you can still use a tracking app to make sure that the foods you choose will get you to your macro targets in the amounts that you consume.

Several different tracking apps are helpful when you follow the macro diet. (See Chapter 7 for some recommendations.) You can use these apps to help create your daily meal plan a day (or more) in advance.

Follow these steps to use an app:

1. Calculate your calorie and macro targets for each meal and snack.

2. Go to your tracking app and input the foods you plan to eat for each meal.

3. Evaluate the numbers and make adjustments as needed so you reach your targets. Add foods, remove foods, or change portion sizes to get where you want to be.

Many apps save the foods that you use frequently, so there is no need to search for a food every time you add it to your meal plan. In addition, some apps allow you to copy and paste from a previous date. These features help to make the meal planning process much more streamlined.

Total tech method

If the thought of doing calculations and planning a menu makes you feel overwhelmed, don't worry. Apps and websites do the whole meal planning process for you — calculations and all!

For example, an app called Prospre generates entire custom meal plans based on your macro targets. And if you don't want to calculate your targets, it'll tackle that task as well. With your targeted numbers, Prospre provides a complete daily menu along with recipes, instructions, and even a grocery list if you prefer. But Propspre isn't the only app or website that provides this service.

TIP

Dozens of meal planning services online and in the app store are specifically targeted to people following a macro diet. Some services require a subscription, while others provide basic services for free with premium services at various price points. Do your homework and research a few before deciding on the best one for you.

The upside to using these apps is that all of the work is done for you. The downside is that the meal plans may not include your favorite foods. If you're unsure if they are right for you, give one of the free services a try for a week and then make a decision about whether it's worth the investment.

Sampling Macro-Balanced Daily Menus

On the next few pages, you'll find daily meal plans for different calorie goals and macro targets. These are not necessarily recommended plans. You should use your personalized calorie and macro targets when putting together your own meal plans. These sample plans are simply provided to give you an idea of how a meal plan might look for different types of people on the macro diet.

Keep in mind that the calorie and macro grams listed are approximate numbers. As I discuss in Chapter 7, even the nutrient data provided by the USDA has a margin of error of up to 20 percent, so numbers may not always add up exactly. But this will not make a significant difference in the success of your plan.

The specific foods you use and your portion sizes will determine your specific grams and calories if you choose to include these meals in your daily plan.

REMEMBER

Don't obsess over every calorie or gram of food on the macro diet. What matters most is that you consume a consistent diet that provides your body with the general balance of nutrition that it needs.

The meal plans listed in this chapter don't include specific recipes or portion sizes. You'll want to adjust those for your own personalized needs. But you can get a sense of what each meal provides in terms of macros and then do the fine-tuning on your own so that you reach your personalized targets.

A 1,500-calorie 40/30/30 meal plan

This is a relatively low-calorie meal plan that someone might follow when trying to lose weight. The plan provides a range of protein sources and would work well for someone who enjoys a wide variety of food, including fruits, vegetables, poultry, and seafood.

You'll notice that the calories are equally divided between each meal so a steady stream of energy is provided throughout the day. Several of the foods, such as the snacks, the chicken lunch, and the salmon can be prepped in advance if you prefer.

» **Breakfast:** 400 calories, 40g carbs, 33g protein, 14g fat

   2-egg omelet with low-fat cheese, spinach, and mushrooms

   Whole grain toast

» **Lunch:** 400 calories, 40g carbs, 33g protein, 14g fat

   Grilled chicken and tossed vegetables with vinaigrette and sunflower seeds

» **Dinner:** 400 calories, 40g carbs, 33g protein, 14g fat

   Roasted Salmon with quinoa and roasted vegetables

» **Snack #1:** 150 calories, 15g carbs, 12g protein, 5g fat

   2 tablespoons hummus + veggie sticks

» **Snack #2:** 150 calories, 15g carbs, 12g protein, 5g fat

   1/2 cup Greek yogurt with 1/4 cup mixed berries and 1/4 c granola

» **TOTALS:** 1,500 calories, 150g carbohydrate, 123g protein, 52g fat

A 1,500-calorie 50/20/30 meat-free meal plan

This is a lower-calorie plan that provides a bit more carbohydrate, a little bit less protein, and roughly the same amount of fat than the plan described in the preceding section. You'll see that this plan provides for more energy earlier in the day and less energy later in the day.

This meal plan might be appealing to someone who wants to cut back on their meat intake. To make this plan fully vegetarian (or vegan), swap the hard-boiled egg for a handful of nuts instead, and grill tofu for dinner instead of shrimp. If you enjoy shrimp, use the Grilled Shrimp Kebobs recipe in Chapter 16.

» **Breakfast:** 428 calories, 61g carbs, 14g protein, 18g fat

   Whole-grain English muffin with peanut butter and banana

» **Lunch:** 591 calories, 111g carbs, 20g protein, 7g fat

   Rice and bean burrito with spinach, shredded carrots, and salsa

» **Dinner:** 328 calories, 12g carbs, 33g protein, 16g fat

   Shrimp and veggie kebobs with red pepper, mushrooms, and onion

>> **Snack #1:** 78 calories, 1g carbs, 6g protein, 5g fat

1 large hard-boiled egg

>> **Snack #2:** 129 calories, 9g carbs, 13g protein, 6g fat

1 cup edamame

>> **TOTALS:** 1,553 calories,194g carbohydrate, 88g protein, 52g fat

An 1,800-calorie 50/25/25 meal plan

This meal plan provides a steady stream of energy throughout the day. It would work well for someone who enjoys a variety of different foods in their diet. You can use the Mixed Berry Smoothie recipe in Chapter 14 if you'd like, which provides a similar nutritional profile.

>> **Breakfast:** 470 calories, 59g carbs, 33g protein, 11g fat

Scrambled egg whites on a whole-wheat bagel with cheddar cheese

>> **Lunch:** 380 calories, 59g carbs, 20g protein, 10g fat

Whole-wheat pasta with peas, carrots, broccoli, and parmesan

>> **Dinner:** 550 calories, 44g carbs, 28g protein, 29g fat

Grilled sirloin steak with basmati rice, roasted bell pepper, zucchini, and yellow squash

>> **Snack:** 400 calories, 40g carbs, 37g protein, 5g fat

Mixed berry protein smoothie

>> **TOTALS:** 1,800 calories, 202g carbohydrate, 118g protein, 55g fat

An 1,800-calorie 33/33/34 meal plan

This meal plan provides macros in relatively equal proportions (with fat slightly higher). It provides plenty of protein at every meal (including dessert!) along with healthy fats, fruits, and vegetables. If you want to cut back on the fat to get the percentage in line with USDA guidelines (less than 30 percent of total daily calories), use non-fat Greek yogurt instead of mayonnaise when you make your tuna salad for lunch.

Check out the recipes for the Cottage Cheese Apple Pancakes (Chapter 15), the Baked Pork Chops with Mashed Cauliflower (Chapter 16) and the Nutty Homemade Protein Bars (Chapter 17). Adjust your portion size for each recipe to meet your personalized macro needs. The meal plans below show how you might pair different recipes for a complete day's worth of eating.

>> **Breakfast:** 400 calories, 36g carbs, 29g protein, 15g fat

Cottage Cheese Apple Pancakes with mixed berries (see recipe in Chapter 15)

Lean turkey breakfast sausage

>> **Lunch:** 650 calories, 42g carbs, 74g protein, 21g fat

Tuna salad sandwich with grapes

>> **Dinner:** 375 calories, 20g carbs, 23g protein, 23g fat

Baked Pork Chops with Mashed Cauliflower (see recipe in Chapter 16) and sauteed green beans

>> **Snack:** 295 calories, 32g carbs, 14g protein, 14g fat

Nutty Homemade Protein Bar (see recipe Chapter 17)

>> **Dessert:** 80 calories, 16g carbs, 6g protein, 0g fat

Greek yogurt frozen fudge bar

>> **TOTALS:** 1,800 calories, 146g carbohydrate, 146g protein, 73g fat

An 1,800-calorie 40/30/30 meal plan

This meal plan provides a range of protein sources and would work well for someone who enjoys a wide variety of food, including fruits, vegetables, poultry, and seafood. You'll notice that the calories are equally divided between each meal so there is a steady stream of energy throughout the day. Several of the foods, such as the snacks, the chicken lunch, and the salmon can be prepped in advance if you prefer.

>> **Breakfast:** 315 calories, 47g carbs, 28g protein, 3g fat

Whole-grain, high-protein cereal, non-fat Greek yogurt, kiwi, and berries

>> **Lunch:** 687 calories, 82g carbs, 63g protein, 14g fat

Mixed grains (wild rice, farro, quinoa) with grilled chicken breast and roasted carrots

» **Dinner:** 627 calories, 37g carbs, 29g protein, 42g fat

Baked halibut with sweet potato fries and asparagus

» **Snack:** 180 calories, 17g carbs, 21g protein, 4g fat

Chocolate protein bar

» **TOTALS:** 1,809 calories, 183g carbohydrate, 141g protein, 63g fat

A 2,000-calorie 50/25/25 meal plan

This meal plan works for someone who needs approximately 2,000 calories per day. It provides about half of the calories from carbohydrates with about 25 percent from protein and about 25 percent from fat. You'll enjoy a hearty lunch with plenty of protein and carbs to fuel a late afternoon workout if that's on your schedule.

Use the recipes for the Super Easy Three Bean Salad (Chapter 16) and the Orange Dreamsicle Smoothie (Chapter 14) if you like this meal plan.

» **Breakfast:** 386 calories, 49g carbs, 11g protein, 17g fat

2 slices avocado toast, with tomato slices and balsamic vinegar

» **Lunch:** 735 calories, 114g carbs, 40g protein, 15g fat

Super Easy Three Bean Salad (see recipe in Chapter 16) and sliced apple

» **Dinner:** 639 calories, 71g carbs, 40g protein, 23g fat

Thai chicken lettuce wraps with white rice and edamame

» **Snack:** 333 calories, 44g carbs, 33g protein, 4g fat

Orange Dreamsicle Smoothie (see recipe in Chapter 14)

» **TOTALS:** 2,093 calories, 278g carbohydrate, 124g protein, 59g fat

A 2,000-calorie, plant-based meal plan

This meal plan provides plenty of fiber and healthy fats to boost satiety (the feeling of fullness). This is a lower protein plan (with just under 20 percent of calories coming from protein). But you can boost the protein grams by adding a plant-based protein powder (such as pea protein or soy protein) to the oatmeal. Swapping quinoa for brown rice in the stir fry will also increase the protein grams a bit.

» **Breakfast:** 400 calories, 57g carbs, 11g protein, 17g fat

Oatmeal with almond milk, chia seeds, and banana

» **Lunch:** 700 calories, 111g carbs, 30g protein, 16g fat

Quinoa salad with mixed greens, chickpeas, veggies, and balsamic dressing

» **Dinner:** 525 calories, 62g carbs, 23g protein, 23g fat

Vegan stir fry with tofu, brown rice, broccoli, zucchini, bell peppers, and mushrooms

» **Snack #1:** 150 calories, 15g carbs, 12g protein, 5g fat

2 tablespoons hummus with carrot and celery sticks

» **Snack #2:** 225 calories, 28g carbs, 3g protein, 12g fat

A handful of grapes and a square (1 ¼" square by ¼" thick) of dark chocolate

» **TOTALS:** 2,000 calories, 273g carbohydrate, 79g protein, 73g fat

4

Overcoming Obstacles

Nurture motivation and build a network of support so that you feel inspired to reach your goals.

Enjoy restaurant dining, travel, and social occasions while keeping your macro diet plan on track.

Decide if you want to drink alcoholic beverages while tracking your macros and figure out how to count those calories.

IN THIS CHAPTER

» Finding and using different types of motivation

» Connecting with the macro diet community for support

» Getting encouragement from family and friends

» Implementing strategies to stay on track when times get tough

Chapter 11

Finding Support and Motivation

A t the beginning of any new exercise or nutrition program, it is common to feel excited and inspired. You've got ideas about where your new journey will take you and visions of how success will feel when you reach your goals. Also, at this point in the journey, you probably haven't encountered typical challenges, so you've got no disappointment to drag you down. But this honeymoon phase doesn't last forever.

TIP

Even though you will probably feel highly motivated at the start of the macro diet, you can expect to encounter challenges along the way. Preparing for these challenges can help you move through them and continue on the path to success.

Typically, challenges arise by the end of the first month of any new habit change. But it can happen even sooner than that. When researchers analyzed patterns related to New Year's resolutions, they found that most people dump their commitment within a month, and about one in four people don't even make it one week.

The trick to sticking with your diet is to try to harness that early-stage enthusiasm so that you can turn to it when the newness of the diet starts to wear off. In this chapter, I help you determine what's hindering your motivation so you can address it effectively. I explain how to look within yourself for inspiration and how to turn to others for motivation as well. I provide ideas for getting support from family and friends, and finally, I give you some ideas for what to do when you feel overwhelmed and want to give up.

Identifying the Barriers

So, what barriers can you expect to encounter? The issues that arise will vary from person to person, but they generally fall into one of three categories: physical, environmental, or emotional. In some cases, if you can view the barrier as a challenge rather than an obstacle standing in the way of success, you can use it as an opportunity for growth and move past it.

Physical barriers

Physical barriers include issues that relate to your general well-being or a medical diagnosis. For instance, if you're taking a medication that affects your weight, it will be much harder for you to lose weight. Physical barriers might also include issues like fatigue, discomfort, dehydration, or lack of sleep.

Any issue that affects your physical well-being can play a role in your nutritional needs and in your food choices. So, it is important to address physical barriers early in the macro diet process so they don't impede your progress.

REMEMBER

It's always smart to check with your healthcare provider before making any significant dietary change. This is especially true if you have an underlying medical issue. If you're experiencing other physical barriers, you can discuss those as well. Your provider may be able to help you address sleep issues or other concerns that affect your health or your ability to be successful on the macro diet.

Environmental barriers

Environmental barriers are those that involve your surroundings, such as your home or your workspace. If your environment doesn't support a healthy diet and exercise plan, it can feel like you're constantly climbing a mountain in order to get healthy.

Environmental barriers can include problems like limited access to healthy food or to exercise facilities, poor social support, or a lack of time due to social, family, and professional pressures.

Before going on the macro diet, you may want to take some time to evaluate your environment to see if you can make changes to stack the odds in your favor.

For instance, if you don't feel like you have time to make healthy meals, then visit Chapter 8 and learn to prep healthy meals in advance. That way, when you're short on time (and probably tired), you have a macro-balanced meal ready to go.

If your new macro diet plan will involve exercise, think about how and where you will work out. Is there a gym on the way to your workplace? Do you have exercise equipment at home? Can you incorporate physical activity into your daily routine (such as biking to work or walking during your lunch break)?

If you aren't sure where to buy healthy food in your area, can you use online services that provide grocery delivery? Can you talk to your local grocer about getting more foods that align with your meal plan?

REMEMBER

The more convenient it is to stick to your goals, the more likely you are to reach them. So, take steps to set up your environment for success before starting on your macro diet journey.

Emotional barriers

Emotional or psychological barriers can include skepticism about your ability to reach your goals, high stress levels, or simply a lack of motivation.

Emotional barriers are very common when you attempt any type of habit change, but they are exceptionally common with diet changes related to weight loss. For instance, you might find yourself facing one of these issues on your journey to lose weight.

>> **All-or-nothing thinking** occurs when you view your eating habits as a complete success or a total failure. For instance, if you don't hit your macros one day and beat yourself up because of it. This type of thought pattern can be tough on you mentally and might make it hard for you to return to your program after you deviate from it or enjoy an unscheduled indulgence. If you find yourself practicing all-or-nothing thinking, remember that the macro diet is a plan about finding balance, not perfection. Seeking perfect compliance to any macro number (or any diet) is simply not attainable or realistic.

>> **Negative body image** can impact your mental health, especially if you tie your body image to your self-worth. You might put yourself at risk for a negative body image if you spend time comparing yourself to unrealistic images on social media. Staying off of social media is one way to manage this barrier, but in some cases, seeking the help of a behavioral health specialist may be warranted.

WARNING

Making any dietary changes in order to conform to perceived social or external standards about body appearance is unhealthy and should be addressed before going on this or any diet.

>> **Stress** is (unfortunately) part of our everyday lives, but it can wreak havoc on a weight loss plan. Many of us turn to food for comfort when we experience stress. The key to confronting this challenge is to explore new ways to manage stress relief, such as massage, meditation, journaling, or simply connecting with supportive friends.

If your thought patterns or mental well-being are standing in the way of success on the macro diet, take a step back to evaluate.

TIP

If you find yourself practicing negative self-talk or experiencing negative emotions connected to food or eating, consider reaching out to a therapist or other mental health professional.

Putting yourself on solid ground emotionally before you start making dietary changes will help ensure that you reach your goals in a sustainable and healthy way.

Understanding the Two Types of Motivation

Behavioral health specialists have identified two different kinds of motivation: intrinsic and extrinsic. Each type of motivation can be harnessed to reach your goals.

>> **Extrinsic motivation** comes from external sources.

>> **Intrinsic motivation** comes from within.

One type of motivation isn't necessarily better than the other. But it's important to understand how each type is used. In different circumstances each type of motivation can be helpful.

Extrinsic motivation

When you're extrinsically motivated, your desire to carry out a task or a goal comes from outside of yourself. Your motivation is external. That is, you hope to gain a reward or avoid a punishment.

For example, you probably remember completing household chores as a kid because your parents told you to. You may have completed the chores out of a sense of obligation, not because you actually enjoyed washing the dishes or mowing the lawn. Therefore, you were extrinsically motivated.

Extrinsic motivation sometimes gets a bad rap, but it is not always a negative thing. Sometimes, a little external pressure is helpful when you need to do something that you don't enjoy.

For instance, you might have a school assignment or a work task that is due. To get it done, you promise yourself a relaxing afternoon of watching your favorite movie when the assignment is completed. In that case, extrinsic motivation is helpful in the short term.

But studies have shown that this type of motivation is usually not sufficient to promote long-term adherence to any significant behavior change, like a diet. In addition, extrinsic pressure — like the pressure you might feel to conform to social pressures about how to look — can lead to unhealthy behaviors, such as binge eating or other unhealthy eating behaviors.

For instance, if you want to use the macro diet to slim down because you want to look more like your favorite influencer on Instagram, then your motivation is extrinsic. In these situations, however, extrinsic pressure can be stress-inducing and is likely to backfire in the long run.

If your motivation to follow the macro diet is extrinsic, especially if it relates to changing your appearance to conform to unrealistic standards on social media, then the program is not likely to be successful in the long term and may even be harmful to your well-being.

WARNING

If you feel social pressure to look a certain way or have a certain body size, reach out to a behavioral health professional who specializes in body image issues. You can enjoy a healthful diet and support good nutrition without the stress that social media and other forms of social pressure can induce.

Intrinsic motivation

When you make a behavioral change because you feel inspired from within, you're taking advantage of intrinsic motivation.

Intrinsic motivation happens when you do something out of the simple joy or sense of reward that it brings to you. If you enjoy a particular challenge or gain a sense of accomplishment from an activity, then you're intrinsically inspired.

REMEMBER

When it comes to changing your diet, intrinsic motivation is your key to success. Multiple studies have shown that when people are able to tap into intrinsic motivation, they are more likely to stick with an activity or stay on track with a goal for the long-term.

So how do you harness the power of intrinsic motivation? Use these tips to tap into yours:

1. **Revisit your SMART goal.** You may have articulated your internal motivation when you set your SMART goal (read Chapter 5 if you haven't set a goal yet). The "R" in SMART refers to *relevant*. In setting your goal, you wrote down why this goal was meaningful to you. Remind yourself of the reasons that you decided to change your diet in the first place.

2. **Discover and emphasize joy.** Think about what you enjoy about your new meal plan. Can you add your favorite foods to your daily diet? Are there any new skills that you look forward to mastering? Are you giving yourself credit for each new accomplishment that you tackle? Keeping a journal can help you work through ideas and allows you the space to acknowledge your successes.

3. **Connect with others.** Sharing your experiences with like-minded individuals is a great way to boost validation and motivation. Connecting with others can be especially impactful if the people in your immediate circle aren't on board with your macro diet journey. It can also be a great way to share tips and ideas or get help with challenges. (See "Finding the Macro Diet Community.")

Keep in mind that the presence of extrinsic motivators can sometimes hinders the fostering of intrinsic motivation.

External rewards can create a distraction that might stand in the way of you listening to your internal voice. Therefore, if you're having a hard time finding your internal motivation, you may need to remove external rewards.

For instance, if you always reward yourself at the end of the week with a trip to your favorite restaurant, you might be shortchanging yourself from feeling the quiet sense of accomplishment that comes with successfully completing another week. The more you can tune into those feelings and celebrate their presence, the more you encourage that internal inspiration that is likely to keep you motivated for the long term.

Finding the Macro Diet Community

The popularity of the macro diet has exploded in recent years, leading to a rise in communities that share their ideas and experiences. So, you won't have to look very far to find people to connect with.

WARNING

You may need to exercise a bit of caution, however, because not all of these groups foster healthy attitudes about nutrition, body image, or weight. Also, since the macro diet is not a branded or commercial diet, no single owner or company is behind it. Therefore, people who use social media may use macro diet hashtags to post unrelated or even inappropriate content online.

You're likely to find most groups through social media, your gym, and through paid services. I explain how each type works so you can explore on your own.

On social media

The great thing about social media is that it allows you to expand your world with a few simple clicks of a keyboard or smartphone. So, if you live in a small town or in an area where it is hard for you to find people with similar interests, you have the opportunity to find them online for free.

TIP

Instagram, TikTok, Threads, and Facebook all have robust communities that celebrate the macro diet. You can find them by searching keyword phrases such as macros, macro diet, macro tracking, track your macros, or flexible diet.

You might also try searching "IIFYM," which stands for "if it fits your macros."

You should exercise some caution when choosing which communities to join. Recent studies have suggested that even when online influencers use body-positive language or hashtags in their posts, they might still push unrealistic standards related to body size.

For instance, according to one study, certain "fitspiration" accounts (such as those using the "fitspo" hashtag) often promote images of very thin or very lean fitness models and promote unhealthy or unrealistic body shapes.

If you enjoy social media, use it to connect with others and find inspiration on your macro diet journey. Just take some time to explore various communities before you jump in head first.

At your gym or workout hive

If exercise is a key component of your macro diet experience, then you can probably find fellow macro trackers at your gym or health club.

You may be able to connect with others simply by chatting with others after a class or in the weight room. If you're part of a running or cycling group, start up a conversation before a workout.

Find out if your health club offers any classes or other resources devoted to nutritional wellness. Talk to a personal trainer, group fitness instructor, or gym manager about opportunities, and if none are currently available, suggest starting a class or a meet-up group.

Through free or paid online services

Nutrition websites and weight-loss companies might provide macro tracking support and services for free or for a subscription fee. For example, Precision Nutrition provides several free services to help you track your macros, such as a macro calculator. If you decide that you want more support, the website also offers group or one-on-one coaching with a certified nutrition professional for a fee.

You'll also find well-known weight-loss companies and smaller nutritional coaching services online that offer programs to help you follow the macro diet.

Some online coaching services are actually artificial intelligence (AI) generated responses that might be helpful but may not give you the personal coaching that you need.

Do a little research before investing in any service to save yourself from hassle and disappointment. Find out exactly what you get for your fee and find out who is offering the support.

Enlisting the Help of Family and Friends

Do you change your eating habits when you're around your family or friends? Some studies suggest that we do. This can impact the success of your macro experience if you spend a lot of time in social situations or with family.

Research suggests that we tend to change the *amount* of food we eat and the *type* of food we eat to match the choices made by our closest companions in social environments.

So, it makes sense to enlist the support of family and friends when you're trying to change your dietary habits. You can approach this situation in several ways to get the encouragement you need:

» **Get vocal.** Share your goals with the people whom you admire. Tell them why this dietary change is important to you and how you plan to tackle your new meal plan. If you're using an app to track your macros, show them how it works. You may even want to brag a little bit about a recent success. Your people are more likely to support your goals if they understand them better.

» **Be specific.** Your friends or family might want to help, but they may not know how. The more specific you can be with them, the more likely you'll be to get what you need. For instance, you might ask someone to help with childcare on the day when you do food prep. That way, you can get your shopping and cooking done with less stress. Or maybe you have a family member who is a pro in the kitchen. If your kitchen skills are lacking, ask them to give you a lesson or two.

» **Monitor stress.** Let's face it, family gatherings can be fun and exciting. But sometimes they are also stressful. If you tend to eat (or overeat) to manage stress, then family gatherings have the potential to derail your diet. So, try to come up with an alternate stress-relief method. Take a walk or connect with a supportive family member when things start to get hairy.

Also, remember that the macro diet is a *flexible* diet. You can choose to backburner your food plan for a special event.

TIP

If you have an important family event or social occasion, ditch your diet for the night. Taking a day off isn't going to make a significant difference in your long-term results.

The bottom line is that your friends and family are likely to support you if they understand how important this habit change is to you and if they understand that their influence matters. Be clear with your needs, and you're likely to get the support and inspiration you need.

Staying on Track When Motivation Hits the Road

Even with strong intrinsic motivation, short-term extrinsic motivation, and support from family and friends, challenges can still arise from time to time. Life intervenes, and factors like work, school, or family matters take priority. Sticking to *any* diet may seem overwhelming. At times like these, you may feel like throwing in the towel.

TIP

You will experience moments when the hassle of maintaining your macro program seems to outweigh any benefit of sticking to the diet. If you can have a backup plan in place, you're far more likely to get back on track and reach your long-term goals.

You can use a few different strategies when your motivation tanks. Consider these options and choose whatever plan you think will be easiest to navigate (which might also include a combination of all three).

Using intermittent tracking

If you're tracking all of your meals and snacks successfully, you're most likely to see health, weight, and athletic performance benefits. But it is also a lot of work. If life gets hectic, start practicing occasional or intermittent tracking.

To implement intermittent tracking, choose one meal per day to target and track those macros. Or choose two or three days during the week when you shoot for macro-balanced meals.

If budget allows, this is also a great time to invest in meal delivery services that offer macro-balanced meals. Or if you have a family member who cooks, ask for their support and give them meal prep recipes to assemble for you.

The bottom line is that you can stick to your program without the work of tracking every single meal. Simply do as much as you can until you have the time and the bandwidth to tackle more.

Prepping foods instead of meals

Another way to scale back slightly without throwing in the towel is to prep foods instead of full meals. Choose a few foods that you enjoy and that are easy to prep and store. For instance, make a batch of hard-boiled eggs. Chop up some carrot sticks, celery stalks, or jicama and keep them in the fridge with a tub of hummus. You can even buy them pre-cut if that is easier. Thaw some precooked shrimp and keep them in the refrigerator with a few slices of lemon.

TIP

Keeping healthy, easy-to-grab foods is a great way to support a balanced diet without the work of cooking or prepping entire meals.

You can grab these quick foods when you need a snack or to help balance out a meal. Just making small choices that support your nutritional goals can help you to feel like you're still on track with your goals.

Building macro meals on the fly

If you're away from home when challenges hit, sticking to your program may feel especially challenging. Or perhaps you're home but have no time to cook or prep meals. You can still make smart choices and maintain good nutrition.

In Chapter 16, I go over the basics of building macro-balanced meals. You can use the same strategies that I mention there when you're on the road or short on time. You won't be weighing foods or calculating grams of macros, but you can still assemble a meal that supports good health.

Just follow these basic steps:

1. **Choose a protein.** A typical 3-ounce serving of most protein sources is about the size of a deck of cards. If you want two servings, shoot for two decks of cards. Keep in mind that if you're eating at a restaurant, your protein will likely be 2 to 3 servings.

2. **Add healthy carbs.** Choose green leafy or cruciferous vegetables (Brussels sprouts, spinach, broccoli) to add to your plate (if possible), and then fill in the rest of the space with grains or starchy veggies.

3. **Let fat happen.** You usually don't have to worry about adding fat because oils are often used in cooking and preparing protein, veggies, and grains. There might also be fats in salad dressings or in other sauces.

Simply building a plate around your three macros can help you to get balanced nutrition to support good health. You can get back to tracking grams and macros when you have time.

REMEMBER

Most importantly, give yourself credit for creating and implementing a backup plan. The more you tackle challenges head-on, the greater your confidence will become. Simply taking small steps to stay on track will make a big difference over the long term.

Chapter **12**

Sticking to the Macro Diet When Eating Away from Home

t is usually a good idea to start the macro diet when your life is, well, . . . *boring*. That is, it's best to begin when your life is as typical as possible. You don't want any vacations, big work projects, or major life events to distract you from focusing on building a nutrition plan that works for you.

By starting the macro diet when your life is fairly routine — your schedule is predictable, and there are no major stressors going on — you give yourself the opportunity to begin on a solid foundation.

Those early weeks will give you time to see how different meal schedules and macro balances support your typical daily workload. Then you can make adjustments as needed based on your schedule and your personalized needs.

But eventually, life will intervene. There will be parties to attend, important assignments due at work or school, vacations to enjoy, and all sorts of other disruptions to your routine. When these occasions pop up, you'll have the opportunity to decide if you'd like to take a short break from your macro plan or if you want to stick to it while you manage your other event.

TIP

In this chapter, I show you how to navigate the various interruptions that might come along when you are tracking your macros. I give you easy-to-follow advice for daily life (including workplace eating tips), various ways to manage social occasions, and expert guidance for managing restaurants and travel.

When to Take a Break from the Macro Diet (or not!)

You can always take a break from the macro diet for a day, a week, or longer to suit your needs. This diet is called the flexible diet because you can modify it at any time and for any reason.

Asking yourself these questions might help you to determine the best course of action for you:

>> **How long of a break will I need?** If you simply want to take an evening off to enjoy a restaurant meal without counting macros, then do it! You don't want the macro diet to interfere with life's enjoyable moments. If you defer to the diet too often, it will eventually become unsustainable.

On the other hand, if you have a regular recurring event, like a weekly book group dinner at a restaurant, you may want to make a plan to keep that night's meal in line with the dietary goals you've set for yourself.

>> **How often will this event recur?** Are you going on a once-in-a-lifetime vacation? Then don't worry about your diet! Savor the experiences and the flavors that your destination has to offer. You don't want *any* diet (except one that is required for medical reasons) to interfere with such an experience.

On the other hand, if you are required to travel once per month for work, then coming up with a sustainable way to manage that time away from home will help you to stay on track over the long term.

>> **Can the macro diet support me during this event?** Perhaps you started the macro diet while you were training for an out-of-town marathon. You want to enjoy local food and festivities at your race destination, but you also want to set a personal record (PR) at the event. In this case, sticking to the diet would make more sense, at least until after race day.

>> **Am I willing to go back to counting my macros after my event?** This question is less about your special occasion and more about the sustainability of the diet itself. If you find yourself looking for special events to use as an excuse to ditch the diet for a day (or longer), then you should revisit your plan and make adjustments.

Taking a break from the macro diet is perfectly fine. In fact, it can even be a good thing! But if you find yourself needing a break on a regular basis, then you should revisit your goal, reconfigure your macro targets, and make the diet more enjoyable so that you can sustain it without feeling deprived.

Tips for Work and Daily Life

As you get settled into your macro diet routine, you'll need to experiment with different tracking strategies, meal plans, and schedules to find out what works best. Take plenty of time to build a solid foundation.

In the early weeks of the macro diet, start small and build slowly as you gain confidence and see results. If you get frustrated, don't be afraid to dial it back to gain your footing.

For example, if tracking macros for three meals per day becomes too time-consuming, focus on tracking just one main meal each day. As you get more efficient, you might (or might not!) choose to track macros for other meals.

These tips and hacks for home and work life also can help you to enjoy meals and stick to whatever nutritional goals you've set for yourself.

Keep an organized kitchen

Have a thoughtful plan for your pantry and cabinets. Keep macro-friendly foods on the shelves that are easiest to reach and that you see most often. Move foods that you want to consume sparingly to the highest or lowest shelves so it takes a little extra effort to get to them. Then if you find yourself grazing, you'll see the most nutritious items first.

Pack your lunch after dinner

Prepare the next day's lunch after you finish dinner. You're likely to make smarter and more nutritious decisions about your meal when your belly is full and you feel satiated.

Dine like you're at a restaurant (even when you're at home)

Slow down your eating experience at home to increase enjoyment. First, serve your salad on a small plate. Then enjoy your entrée on a separate plate. Try not to leave large serving bowls on the table.

TIP

When you take more time to eat, you give your belly a chance to recognize the signs of satiety (fullness). This may help you to feel more satisfied after eating.

Avoid eating at your desk

On some days, you may feel tempted to work through lunch and dine at your desk. But studies suggest that taking a break can help boost productivity, and it will certainly help you to enjoy your meal more fully. Go outside if weather permits, or even take a short respite to go to a dining area or breakroom.

TIP

Creating a designated meal "environment" may help you to use mindful eating techniques such as immersing yourself in the smell, taste, and texture of your food and savoring every bite.

Enjoy a post-meal mint

If you are a person who tends to continue eating after you're full, try popping a mint in your mouth when you want to be done. The cool refreshing flavor helps to put a "stop" to the eating cycle. Some people also brush their teeth after dinner for this same reason (and for good dental hygiene!).

TIP

If you like to graze after eating and consume mindless calories, having a mint after meals might be a helpful hack. You might also try drinking a cup of mint tea to calm your mind and taste buds.

Delegate dish duty

Another helpful tip for post-meal nibblers is to delegate dish duty to someone else (or postpone doing the dishes if you live alone). It's easy to pick away at food if you're in the kitchen after mealtime is complete. Sometimes the smartest thing to do is to get out of the kitchen until your interest in food has subsided.

Go for a walk after eating

You're not going to want to engage in vigorous activity after eating, but if you can go for a walk, you'll be doing your body a favor. Some studies have suggested that a post-meal walk can help to lower blood pressure. Several small studies have also suggested that walking after a meal may the best way to manage high sugar spikes (called *post-prandial glycemic response*) after a carb-rich meal. Plus, taking time to enjoy some fresh air is sure to help relieve stress.

Simple Strategies for Special Occasions

So many social occasions revolve around eating. Whether it is a special family meal, a birthday party, a tailgate party before the big game, or simply a meet-up among friends, we often plan and gather around food. This can make macro tracking tricky — especially when the foods offered are not foods that you are familiar with.

TIP

The easiest way to manage these situations is simply to enjoy the meal and don't worry about your macros. One meal isn't going to make a big difference.

But you may want to stick to your plan. For instance, if you've set a calorie goal for weight loss, you don't want to overeat, and you know you have a habit of nervous snacking in social situations. In those scenarios, you can use these tips to stick to a healthy eating plan.

Bring a dish

If you are going to an event and you're unsure if the food offerings will align with your plan, offer to bring a dish. Then prepare something that you enjoy that will boost your macro plan and help keep your diet on track. For some beginner-friendly recipes, check out Chapters 16 and 17, where you'll find recipes for appetizers (snacks), desserts, or main dishes. Each recipe provides a balance of macros for you and your friends or family to enjoy.

Get chatty

You probably remember learning this rule of basic table etiquette as a child: Don't talk with your mouth full. So, one way to avoid mindless nibbling is to engage in conversation. You'll spend more time getting to know new friends and acquaintances and less time eating.

Stand away from the food

Another strategy to avoid mindless snacking is to situate yourself away from the food table. Offer to help the host with greeting guests or taking coats. Circulate and meet new people. If it's a casual outdoor event, start an activity like tossing a football or a frisbee.

Ways to Enjoy Healthy Restaurant Dining

Eating out has gotten easier in recent years for people who follow special diets. More and more restaurants are offering plant-based options, gluten-free options, and choices for people who don't eat certain foods, like dairy. And some restaurants now provide nutrient information on the menu, making macro tracking much easier.

This section shares some tricks to help you stick to a healthy eating plan when dining out.

Plan ahead

If possible, look up the restaurant's menu online before you go. You'll be able to get an idea of the healthier options available, which allows you the time to make a more informed choice. If nutrient information is available, you may be able to track your macros before your meal to keep your program on track.

Practice mindful eating

Mindful eating practices are those habits that help you to enjoy the sight, smell, and texture of the dining experience to maximize enjoyment. Researchers have found that focusing on mindful eating in restaurants can help you to increase food satisfaction with smaller portion sizes.

TIP

The simplest way to practice mindfulness in a restaurant is to eat slowly and engage all of your senses. Enjoy the presentation of your plate, the restaurant environment, the various smells, and the taste and texture of each bite.

Eat by a window

Another way to increase enjoyment and encourage healthy eating in a restaurant is to sit by a window — especially if the view allows you to enjoy nature. Exposure to trees, grass, and other greenery helps to decrease stress and improve mood, which may help you to make healthier, feel-good food decisions.

Learn menu lingo

If you're looking for leaner protein options on the menu, search for entrees that are "grilled," "baked," "steamed," or "roasted." These preparation methods usually use less fat than options that are described as "crispy," "fried," "creamy," "battered," or "smothered." (Even though something smothered in a creamy sauce may sound delicious.)

If any of the lingo is unclear, just ask. Your server will be able to decode any jargon so you can make decisions that align with your goals.

Ask for modifications

Most restaurants are more than happy to make slight variations to menu items. For instance, you might ask for steamed veggies or a salad instead of chips or fries with a sandwich. Or you might request that sauce or dressing be served on the side.

REMEMBER

You are the paying customer, so asking (politely) for slight modifications is perfectly acceptable.

Recommendations for Enjoying Macro-Friendly Travels

The fact that the macro diet is a flexible diet allows you the room to take time off when you'd like. So, if you've planned a special getaway with your partner and you don't want to worry about balancing your macros while you are away, then don't do it!

TIP

There is nothing wrong with taking time "off" from your eating plan. In fact, taking a short break may help with long-term sustainability.

But if you want to stick to some variation of the macro diet while traveling, consider these different ways to enjoy your travel while maintaining your nutritional goals.

Research local food

Do a little research before you go. Learn more about local cuisine and popular dishes at your vacation destination. This can help you estimate the macros of the food you're likely to encounter.

Take plenty of pics

You may not want to track macros during your dining experience. Instead, use the camera on your phone to take pictures of the meals you enjoy while on the road. Then use the images like a photo diary so you can remember what you ate and track your macros later during.

Pick one macro to focus on

Tracking all three macros may be more than you want to handle on vacation. Instead, prioritize one macro and don't worry about the other two. For many macro trackers, this macro will be protein. Remember, protein is essential for maintaining muscle mass, and it also helps to keep you feeling full and satiated. Build your meals around protein as the main component and then add carbs and fat to round out the meal.

Stay hydrated

Drink plenty of fluids to stay hydrated and energized. Staying hydrated may also help to keep hunger at bay.

TIP Sometimes, thirst can be mistaken for hunger, leading to unnecessary eating.

Also, caffeinated and alcoholic beverages dehydrate the body, so balance out those beverages with extra water when possible.

Stay active with joyful activity

If you have paired your macro diet with an exercise plan, you may feel obligated to get in a workout when you're on the road. While there is nothing wrong with that, it's also okay to take some time off from your regular routine.

Try to engage in physical activities that are unique to your destination and that you enjoy. Try kayaking, paddleboarding, hiking, or an urban walk. See if there are cycling expeditions or other active sightseeing opportunities. The extra movement will help offset any indulgences that you enjoy and will help to keep you feeling energized.

Chapter **13**

Consuming Alcohol on the Macro Diet

I f you're like millions of Americans, you enjoy a glass of wine, a beer, or an alcoholic cocktail every now and then. According to the Centers for Disease Control (CDC), you would be considered a moderate drinker if you limit your alcohol intake to two drinks or less per day for a man or one drink or less per day for a woman. Heavy drinking is defined as consuming more than 7 drinks per week for women and more than 14 drinks per week for men.

It is important to understand, however, that any habit of regular drinking can affect your results on the macro diet. This doesn't mean that you must give up alcohol while you're counting and tracking macros. This diet is called "the flexible diet" because you can (and should!) enjoy the foods and beverages that you like while you're following it. But it is also important to understand the role that alcohol can play in the way that your body functions and performs.

In this chapter, I explain how drinking alcohol affects your metabolism, how it changes the way that your body processes both macronutrients and micronutrients, and how drinking might affect your nutritional and performance results. Then I show you how to track calories when you do consume alcohol so you can keep moving toward your goals on the macro diet.

How Alcohol Affects Metabolism

Alcohol is sometimes called "the fourth macro" because it can't be categorized as a carbohydrate, a protein, or a fat. Even though an alcoholic beverage can contain one or more of those macros, the alcohol itself is different.

REMEMBER

Alcohol is calorically dense. While carbohydrates and protein each provide 4 calories per gram, alcohol provides 7 calories per gram.

Fat is also calorically dense. In fact, it provides more calories per gram than alcohol, but fat provides important benefits to the body — such as insulation and nutrient absorption. Alcohol does not.

REMEMBER

Your body can't use calories from alcohol for important bodily functions in the same way that it can use calories from protein, fat, and carbs.

Also, your body has no place to store alcohol calories and the byproducts of alcohol metabolism are toxic to the body, so it works hard to get rid of them as quickly as possible. As a result, your body prioritizes alcohol metabolism over the metabolism of other macros. And it is not just macronutrient metabolism that falls behind. Your body also has a harder time processing and absorbing micronutrients.

REMEMBER

When you drink, the processing of other nutrients (including vitamins and minerals) takes a backseat, and alcohol becomes the driver.

Regardless of how much you drink, the body can only metabolize a certain amount of alcohol every hour. The amount varies significantly from person to person and depends on a range of factors, such as your body size.

Because the way that your body metabolizes alcohol is unique, some people are at a higher risk for alcohol problems than others who may feel fewer harmful effects from alcohol consumption.

The Impact of Alcohol on the Macro Diet

Even though your metabolism is affected by drinking alcohol, an occasional beer or glass of wine isn't likely to have a significant effect on your long-term diet plan. But as drinking frequency increases, so does the likelihood of a negative impact on your overall macro diet success.

REMEMBER

The bottom line is that you won't get the benefits of eating a balanced macro diet if your body is busy metabolizing alcohol. And a hangover (if you drink excessively) carries its own set of consequences.

The primary effects of a hangover can include electrolyte imbalance, hypoglycemia (low blood sugar), stomach irritation, and sleep problems. All of these conditions can affect your ability to perform at your best and make good dietary choices.

As you make decisions about drinking or about drinking frequency, think about the different ways that it might affect your success on the macro diet.

Drinking makes weight loss harder

Adding empty calories to your diet might make losing weight more challenging if your primary goal for the macro diet is weight loss.

Drink calories add up quickly! You have to take into account not just the calories from alcohol (at 7 calories per gram) but also any other calories contained in your drink. A single beverage can contribute hundreds of empty calories to your daily totals.

Furthermore, it is not uncommon to make poor food choices when we're drinking. For instance, would you normally order cheese fries and a pizza at 1 a.m., or is that the booze talking? Studies have suggested that as booze intake increases, diet quality decreases.

But keep in mind that drinking is not necessarily a surefire path to weight gain. When researchers have studied drinking, they often find mixed results.

TECHNICAL STUFF

Moderate drinking is not necessarily linked to weight gain, and researchers can't say for certain that drinking leads to obesity, but in one published report, study authors wrote, "It is reasonable to say that alcohol intake may be a risk factor for obesity in some individuals, likely based on a multitude of factors."

Alcohol can mess with your hormones

Heavy drinking may increase cortisol levels in the body. Cortisol is a hormone produced by the adrenal glands that helps regulate your body's response to stress. Cortisol plays an important role in the body, but chronically high levels have been associated with weight gain, muscle weakness, fragile bones, and other problems.

Heavy drinking (especially when it is chronic) can also have a negative effect on testosterone levels in men. Testosterone is considered to be the "sex hormone" because it helps to regulate libido in men, but it also plays a role in maintaining bone density, body fat distribution, muscle strength, and muscle mass. So having healthy levels is important.

But it is not just men who pay the price for drinking. Women's hormones can be affected as well. In pre-menopausal women even mild-to-moderate alcohol use may disrupt normal menstrual cycling by messing with both estrogen and testosterone levels. And in post-menopausal women, some researchers have linked heavy drinking with poor bone health due to hormonal disruptions. (But strong scientific evidence is lacking in this area because doing controlled studies that involve heavy drinking presents ethical issues.)

A big night out might make workouts less effective

Having one too many drinks can seriously impact workout performance in the day (or days) after your night out. You probably won't be able to work out as hard as you would if you had not consumed alcohol or if you consumed in moderation.

Research has shown an approximate 11 percent decrease in aerobic capacity in those exercising with a hangover. And that's not all. If alcohol is still in your system, you won't get the energy you need to fuel your workout. Remember, the body prioritizes alcohol metabolism while backburning the metabolism of carbohydrates and fat, which are the preferred energy sources during endurance exercise.

So, what if you wait until after your workout to imbibe? You're still not doing yourself any favors. Alcohol impairs your body's ability to recover properly from exercise.

REMEMBER

Drinking can interfere with the body's ability to replenish glycogen (glucose that is stored in muscles and liver to be used as energy), stimulate muscle protein synthesis (build muscle), and restore a healthy pre-workout fluid balance after exercise.

Alcohol contributes to poor-quality sleep

If you drink before bed, you may not get the good night's rest that you need to feel energized and productive the next day. For many people, this is a surprising consequence of drinking — having a beer or a glass of wine can make you sleepy. But that beverage can affect the quality of your sleep throughout the night.

REMEMBER

Drinking alcohol before bed may help you fall asleep, but it can also disrupt restorative sleep cycles throughout the night, decreasing the overall quality of your rest.

If you exercise, the impact may be even more significant. Not getting enough sleep may impact recovery, energy levels, and overall athletic performance.

Calories from alcohol may displace other (more important) calories

If you include a few alcoholic drinks in your meal plan and you do so while maintaining your calorie and macro balance, you're likely displacing other calories that your body needs to perform important functions — like building muscle. If you have adopted the macro diet to support a weight-training program, this can be problematic.

REMEMBER

When protein-rich foods are displaced with alcohol calories (especially in the hours after exercise), your body doesn't build muscle as effectively.

This can even be the case if you consume extra protein. Researchers have found that alcohol consumption significantly decreases muscle protein synthesis even when adequate protein is consumed.

To Drink or Not to Drink?

As you consider the impact of alcohol on your metabolism and on your macro diet goals, you'll want to weigh the pros and cons of keeping alcohol in your life. Keep in mind that this doesn't have to be an "all or nothing" decision. You may want to quit drinking (or cut back) temporarily and then reassess in a month or so.

"Sober months" have become very popular across Europe and North America. Many drinkers decide to take 1 to 3 months away from alcohol to see how it feels and reset their relationship with drinking.

TIP

If you choose to try a sober month, look online and in the app store for resources. Organizations are devoted to helping people try experiments like a Dry January, Dry July, Sober September, or Sober October.

As a result of quitting temporarily (or permanently) you may experience better sleep, clearer skin, improved productivity, elevated mood, and closer relationships with loved ones.

As you weigh your options, consider some of the benefits and drawbacks of drinking.

Potential advantages of moderate drinking

If you don't currently drink, the reasons given here should not be used as a reason to start. It is important to take the word "advantages" with a grain of salt. Some people might argue that the advantages listed here are not necessarily benefits of drinking, *per se*. I wouldn't necessarily disagree with that.

REMEMBER

These reasons for drinking alcoholic beverages can be achieved through other (more healthful) means. Don't assume that you must drink to gain any of these advantages.

Still, people who enjoy moderate alcohol consumption often do so for one of these reasons.

>> **Stress relief:** Alcohol is commonly used to combat stress — and some research backs up this potential benefit. Some studies have suggested that moderate alcohol consumption can help to relieve stress and that a moderate dose of alcohol after a mental stressor may help you to rebound faster.

>> **Camaraderie:** Alcoholic beverages are commonly served at social functions, and often, people gather for the sole purpose of enjoying a beer or a glass of wine together. Even in fitness settings, it is not uncommon for groups to join together and celebrate the end of a workout with a drink together, as it can have a bonding effect.

>> **Heart health:** Some studies suggest that moderate drinking may have a protective effect on your health. Research has suggested that light to moderate alcohol intake (up to one drink per day for women and one or two drinks per day for men) is associated with a decreased risk for coronary artery disease, congestive heart failure, and stroke. Keep in mind, however, that other research results conflict with these findings, and the topic is widely debated.

You may or may not experience these perks of drinking — and there may be others that you enjoy not on this list. It is important to consider all of the reasons that you enjoy drinking if you're going to make an informed decision about continuing the habit.

WARNING

In making decisions about whether or not to drink, you may want to evaluate your current dependence on the habit. Do you enjoy having a drink to wind down at the end of the day or do you *need* a drink to wind down at the end of the day? If you find that you rely on a drink for any benefit, you may want to evaluate your relationship with alcohol and seek professional guidance.

You should also consider some disadvantages to balance out your final decision.

Potential disadvantages of moderate drinking

The most obvious downside to including alcohol in your new, healthy meal plan is that the calories you consume don't contribute in any way to your body's healthy functioning. Alcohol calories are empty calories.

In addition, consider these other cons of habitual alcohol use:

>> **Reduced muscle gains:** Although research results have been inconsistent, some studies suggest that your ability to build muscle (muscle protein synthesis) is reduced if you have a drink after working out. This drawback seems to affect men more than women.

>> **Reliance on less healthy stress relief methods:** If you get in the habit of ending your day with a celebratory beverage, you may be shortchanging yourself out of healthier ways to relieve stress, like going for a walk, talking to a friend, meditation, or enjoying a healthy meal.

>> **Poor sleep and fatigue:** Having a drink or two before bed may help you *fall* asleep, but it can impede your ability to *stay* asleep and get deep sleep throughout the night. As a result, you may feel sluggish the next day. In some cases, you may even skip a workout or make poor food choices as a result.

>> **Weight gain:** At seven calories per gram, alcohol calories can add up quickly. And while light-to-moderate drinking is not associated with fat gain, some studies have linked heavy drinking to weight gain.

Of course, you may not experience all (or any) of these drawbacks, but it is important to keep them in mind so that you can make a thoughtful and balanced decision about your relationship with alcohol.

How to Track Alcohol Calories on the Macro Diet

If you decide to keep alcoholic drinks in your meal plan, you'll need to decide how to count them in your macro diet. Since calories in alcoholic beverages can be significant, it is important to track them along with your other macros. And even though alcohol is sometimes considered "the fourth macro," you don't need another category to count each day. So many people count alcohol calories as a different macro.

In general, people on the macro diet will count their alcohol calories as carbohydrate calories or fat calories, or both. I recommend, however, that you count those calories as fat calories.

Here's why: You don't want to shortchange yourself out of important carbohydrate calories, especially if you pair your macro diet with an exercise plan. If you're a runner, for instance, you need high-quality carbs for energy to fuel your workouts. If you get into the habit of replacing those carbs with empty alcohol calories, you may find that your workouts suffer (especially if you drink often).

So, to count alcoholic beverages as fat, follow these steps:

1. Find out how many calories are in your drink.

2. Take that number and divide it by 9 (the number of calories per fat gram).

3. The result is the number of grams that you add to your total fat grams for the day.

Keep in mind, that some drinks contain significant carbohydrates (such as frozen margaritas, pina coladas, and other sweet beverages). If that is the case, you may want to count your drink calories as carbs.

If you decide to count your alcohol calories as carbs in your macro diet, you would follow the same steps but divide the number of calories in the drink by 4 instead of 9.

1. Find out how many calories are in your drink.

2. Take that number and divide it by 4 (the number of calories per carb gram).

3. The result is the number of grams that you add to your total carb grams for the day.

Check out Table 13-1 to see the typical number of calories in different alcoholic drinks.

TABLE 13-1

Beverage	Serving Size	Calories	Nutrients (carb/protein/fat)
Beer (light)	12 ounces	95	5.8g/0.9g/0g
Beer	12 ounces	145	12.6g/1.6g/0g
Daquiri	8 ounces	244	31g/.07g/0g
Gin and tonic	8 ounces	207	15g/.01g/0g
Margarita	8 ounces	226	22g/.02g/0g
Moscow mule	8 ounces	210	21g/.01g/0g
Old fashioned	2.5 ounces	176	6.7g/0g/0g
Pina colada	12 ounces	656	85g/1.6g/7.1g
Rum	1.5 ounces	97	0g/0g/0g
Rum and cola	6 ounces	179	13g/0g/0g
Tequila	1.5 ounces	97	0g/0g/0g
Vodka	1.5 ounces	97	0g/0g/0g
Vodka soda	6 ounces	97	0g/0g/0g
Wine (red)	5 ounces	125	3.8g/0.1g/0g
Wine (sparkling)	5 ounces	120	3.8g/0.1g/0g
Wine (white)	5 ounces	121	3.8g/0.1g/0g

Calories in alcoholic beverages can vary significantly, especially when you order drinks at a bar or restaurant. For instance, a glass of wine in a restaurant may be the standard five-ounce pour, but some restaurants may give you a glass with up to eight or nine ounces. Obviously, this will affect the number of calories and the amount of alcohol you consume.

The variation can be even more significant with mixed drinks. For instance, a typical margarita has 226 calories. But in some restaurants, a frozen margarita can exceed that number substantially and may even include ingredients that aren't typically in a margarita. A margarita made at home, on the other hand, may have far fewer calories depending on the amount of alcohol you use and the ingredients (such as fresh lime and soda water instead of a premade mixer).

Whatever drink you make (or order), take your time and enjoy it. Drinking has consequences, but if it plays a positive role in your life and your habit falls in the low-risk or moderate range, then you can savor those beverages on the macro diet.

5
Whipping Up Macro Diet Recipes

Serve up a smoothie for a quick and easy meal on-the-go.

Make a morning meal that sets you up for success.

Prepare hearty lunch and dinner entrees to make your mouth water.

Create delicious desserts and savory snacks that really satisfy.

Master meal-prep like a pro with quick and easy food combos.

Chapter 14

Protein-Packed Smoothies

O ne of the things that many people love about the macro diet is that no foods are off-limits. You can enjoy a wide range of foods for breakfast, lunch, and dinner. But sometimes, even with careful meal planning, hitting your daily macro targets is still a challenge. That's when smoothies can be a lifesaver.

A smoothie is a great way to get the nutrition you need either at home or on the go. Smoothies can be budget-friendly; they are easy to carry; and you can get the macros and calories you need without having to cook or even having to sit down to eat. Sounds perfect, right?

If you're a busy macro tracker on the go, knowing how to make a power-packed protein smoothie can help you reach your targets when life gets hectic.

WARNING

Beware of the potential downsides to relying on smoothies for nutrition. Prepackaged smoothies that you find in some convenience marts or fast-food outlets are often high in calories and contain added sugar. And they may not even provide the important nutrients (especially protein) in the quantities that you need! Yikes.

REMEMBER

Even if you prepare your smoothies at home, it is important to choose your ingredients wisely so that these convenient shakes support your nutritional goals.

In this chapter, I share some of my favorite blends and give you the scoop on key ingredients. These recipes and tips will help you make the best choices when shopping so you have everything on hand to make shakes that support your goals.

Choosing the Best Smoothie Ingredients

You have countless options when it comes to smoothie recipes. But most will include certain basic ingredients. For instance, many contain fruit, like berries or bananas, and some also contain fruit juice. Your shake may also include milk or a milk alternative. Then, to boost the protein grams in your beverage, you will probably also want to have some protein powder on hand (although not every smoothie uses protein powder as the main protein source).

Understanding your options for these ingredients will help you get the most bang for your buck when you make your own power-packed smoothies.

AVOIDING BLENDER BLOW-UPS

The success of your smoothie may depend, in part, on your blender. High-speed, high-power blenders and Bullet blenders won't have any problems with course ingredients like seeds, ice, or large chunks of frozen fruit. But many of these blenders cost hundreds (or even thousands) of dollars. If you have a less powerful kitchen blender, you might run into trouble with chunky, frozen, or hard ingredients. But there is no need to break the bank and buy a new appliance if you don't want to.

To get a creamy, well-blended smoothie with a less powerful appliance, break ingredients like frozen fruit into smaller pieces. You may even want to do this before freezing certain items, like bananas. Use crushed ice, ice chips, or pre-chop ice cubes into smaller pieces before adding to your blender jar. And try putting smaller ingredients in the blender first (like frozen blueberries) and adding larger fruits last (like frozen strawberries).

Fruit and fruit juice

You'll notice that many smoothie recipes contain bananas. This potassium-rich fruit adds both creaminess and sweetness to smoothies, so they are great to have on hand. If you prefer a sweeter shake, wait until your bananas are very ripe before using them. If you don't like bananas, consider using avocado, mango, or soaked cashews to get that same velvety texture. Oats and chia seeds can also be used to get a thick, creamy consistency.

TIP

Fresh fruit, like berries, helps to boost the vitamin content of your smoothies. But if budget is a concern, consider buying frozen fruit instead of fresh. In most cases, it is just as nutritious as fresh fruit.

Many grocers sell big bags of mixed berries, mangoes, and other fruit that you can keep in your freezer for months, so you don't have to worry about the fruit going bad. Canned fruit can also be preserved for longer than fresh fruit.

WARNING

Be sure that the frozen or canned fruit you buy doesn't contain any added sugar. Often, fruit is canned in sweetened syrup, so you may end up consuming far more sugar than you bargained for with this option.

Fruit juice is another staple in which you want to look out for added sugar. Always check the Nutrition Facts label or the ingredients list to make sure you know what you're getting. You might see sugars like fructose or corn syrup added to some products. Also, some juice products add fruit juice concentrate (like apple juice concentrate or grape juice concentrate) to increase the sugar content in the beverage. If you use juice for your smoothies, try to find 100 percent juice with no added ingredients.

If you have the option of choosing between fruit juice and whole fruit in your smoothie, opt for real fruit when you can. Fruit juice doesn't provide fiber. And, remember, fiber is your friend. Fiber is a carbohydrate that helps to give you a feeling of fullness that can keep you feeling satisfied hours after eating.

Milk and milk alternatives

If you visit the dairy section of your local grocer, you're likely to see far more milk alternatives than dairy milk. The popularity of products like almond milk, cashew milk, and oat milk has skyrocketed. But so have myths about their nutritional benefits, especially as compared to cow's milk.

If you are lactose intolerant, have a milk allergy, or simply don't like to consume dairy products, it makes sense to choose a non-dairy "milk" product. But it is also important to keep in mind that many of these products include sweeteners and other additives that you may not want in your diet. Always read the ingredients label so you know exactly what you are consuming with your milk of choice.

One cup of cow's milk provides 8 grams of protein, regardless of the fat content. Soy milk provides about the same amount per cup but may also contain unwanted ingredients like added sugar. Almond milk provides about 1.3 grams of protein per cup, oat milk provides about 2 grams per cup, and rice milk provides less than 1 gram of protein per serving.

REMEMBER

If protein is your priority, dairy milk is often your best bet.

Different types of protein powder

Although you can boost the protein content of your smoothie with ingredients like milk, yogurt, or even beans or oats, protein powder is the easiest way to get those important amino acids to help you build and maintain muscle. But not all protein supplements are created equal.

Protein powder terminology

If you look at protein powder labels, you'll see different terms describing the type of protein contained in the product. They refer to the type of processing used to create the product, which affects the level of protein concentration.

>> **Protein concentrate** usually contains about 60–80 percent protein, with the rest of the calories coming from fat and carbohydrates.

>> **Protein isolate** contains roughly 90–95 percent protein because it goes through additional filtering that removes more fat and carbohydrates.

>> **Protein hydrolysates** are processed even further so your body can absorb the protein more quickly and efficiently. This type of protein powder may be a good choice for those with stomach problems, but because it is a newer option for consumers, fewer studies support its effectiveness.

Many people opt for products made with protein powder isolate because they get carbs and fats from other sources, and they want as much protein as possible in their supplements. Also, protein powder isolate is widely available online and in stores, so you're likely to have more options to choose from in terms of budget and flavor. You may want to try different types of protein powders to see which one works best for you.

Protein powder sources

You'll also find protein supplements derived from different sources. Consider the different options available when choosing the best protein powder for you.

>> **Whey protein** is derived from milk. It is widely considered the most efficient form of protein powder because it is absorbed quickly in the body and has been shown in research studies to be highly effective for muscle protein synthesis — especially when consumed after a workout. But if you are lactose intolerant or have a milk allergy, whey protein is not be a good option for you.

>> **Casein protein** is also derived from milk, but it is absorbed more slowly in the body than whey protein. Rather than consuming casein protein after a workout (when you want amino acids delivered quickly to your muscles), many athletes consume casein protein before bed. Like whey protein, it is not a good choice for those who avoid dairy for health reasons or for those who follow a plant-based diet.

>> **Soy protein** is derived from the soybean and is a popular choice among those who follow a vegan or vegetarian diet. It is easily found in most health food stores. But soy protein contains fewer branched-chain amino acids (BCAAs) than cow's milk. BCAAs are especially important for building and maintaining muscle in the body.

>> **Pea protein** is becoming more and more popular, especially among plant-based eaters. Protein derived from peas is more quickly absorbed than casein protein but not quite as rapidly as whey protein. Pea protein is also a good source of BCAAs.

>> **Egg protein** powder is getting harder and harder to find as other types of protein have become more popular. But this supplement, derived from egg whites, is still favored by those who want a complete protein (containing all nine amino acids) but don't want a milk-derived source.

REMEMBER

As you shop for smoothie foods, remember that there is no "right" or "wrong" ingredient to include. Choose the foods that you enjoy and that align with your nutritional goals.

TIP

If you avoid animal-based products, any of these smoothies can be made vegan or vegetarian by swapping out dairy products for non-dairy alternatives. Just be sure that you choose protein powders that are also plant-based. As you explore these recipes, swap out any ingredients as needed to make them your own.

Creamy Sweet Green Smoothie

PREP TIME: 10 MIN	COOK TIME: NONE	YIELD: 1 SERVING

INGREDIENTS

½ apple

1 cup spinach

½ ripe banana, chopped

¼ ripe avocado, in chunks

½ cup cold water

1 full scoop vanilla protein powder

DIRECTIONS

1 Chop apple into large chunks and toss into a blender.

2 Place banana, avocado, spinach, water, and protein powder into the blender.

3 Blend on high until smooth.

4 Pour into a glass and enjoy!

NOTE: The banana and apple provide plenty of sweetness to this recipe so if you don't have vanilla-flavored protein powder, you can use plain protein powder, and you'll still get a sweet, protein-rich treat.

VARY IT! No avocado on hand? No problem. The avocado adds texture and healthy fat to this recipe, but it doesn't contribute substantially to the flavor. So, you can use 2–3 tablespoons of Greek yogurt, silken tofu, or even your favorite nut butter instead.

NUTRITION TIP: This smoothie provides 8 grams or 29 percent of the recommended daily value (DV) of fiber and 26 percent of your daily value of vitamin C.

PER SERVING: *Calories 257 (From Fat 58); Fat 6g (Saturated 1g); Cholesterol 0mg; Sodium 210mg; Carbohydrate 36g (Dietary Fiber 8g); Protein 18g.*

Peanut Butter Banana Smoothie

| PREP TIME: 10 MIN | COOK TIME: NONE | YIELD: 1 SERVING |

INGREDIENTS

1 large frozen banana

½ cup frozen kale

2 tablespoons peanut butter

½ cup vanilla nonfat Greek yogurt

1 cup nonfat milk or milk alternative

DIRECTIONS

1 Slice frozen banana and add to a blender.

2 Add peanut butter, kale, Greek yogurt, and milk to the blender.

3 Blend on high until smooth.

4 Pour into a glass and garnish with a sprinkle of cinnamon or cocoa powder if you prefer.

TIP: Freeze a batch of bananas in advance so that you always have them on hand when you need them. To do so, peel several bananas and lay them on a cookie sheet. Place them in the freezer for about an hour until they are partially frozen. Then place them in an airtight freezer bag and put them back in the freezer so they are ready to grab when you need them.

VARY IT! Add a half scoop of vanilla protein powder to boost the protein content of this smoothie if you prefer. Looking to decrease your fat intake? Try using peanut butter powder instead of peanut butter. Many brands provide 90 percent less fat and 70 percent fewer calories than traditional peanut butter.

NUTRITION TIP: This smoothie provides 433mg of calcium or 33 percent of the DV to help build stronger bones.

PER SERVING: *Calories 484 (From Fat 153); Fat 17g (Saturated 4g); Cholesterol 5mg; Sodium 311mg; Carbohydrate 61g (Dietary Fiber 6g); Protein 29g.*

Mixed Berry Smoothie

PREP TIME: 10 MIN	COOK TIME: NONE	YIELD: 1 SERVING

INGREDIENTS

½ cup frozen mixed berries

½ frozen banana

1 tablespoon chia seeds

1 scoop vanilla protein powder

1 cup nonfat milk or milk alternative

Mint leaf (optional)

DIRECTIONS

1 Add berries, banana, chia seeds, protein powder, and milk to a blender.

2 Blend on high until smooth.

3 Pour into a glass and garnish with a sprig of mint.

VARY IT! Mixed berries can be easily found in the freezer section of most supermarkets, but if there is a particular fresh berry that you prefer, go ahead and use it instead. Simply add a few ice cubes to the blender to keep the beverage cool and refreshing.

NUTRITION TIP: Berries are rich in antioxidants — compounds that work to reverse cell damage in the body. Choose fresh or frozen blueberries, strawberries, raspberries, or blackberries to take advantage of these healing compounds.

PER SERVING: *Calories 345 (From Fat 56); Fat 6g (Saturated 1g); Cholesterol 5mg; Sodium 318mg; Carbohydrate 47g (Dietary Fiber 10g); Protein 28g.*

Pumpkin Pie Smoothie

PREP TIME: 10 MIN	COOK TIME: NONE	YIELD: 1 SERVING

INGREDIENTS

1 large frozen banana

⅓ cup pure pumpkin puree

1 tablespoon almond butter

½ scoop vanilla protein powder

1 teaspoon pumpkin pie spice

½ cup almond milk

Dollop of whipped cream (optional)

DIRECTIONS

1 Slice frozen banana and add to a blender.

2 Add pumpkin puree, almond butter, protein powder, pumpkin pie spice, and almond milk to the blender.

3 Blend on high until smooth.

4 Pour into a glass, top with whipped cream if you'd like, and enjoy.

TIP: You can use fresh pumpkin puree if you have it on hand, but the canned variety works well, too. Just be sure to check the label and avoid those with added ingredients such as added sugar. If you look for pure pumpkin puree (rather than pumpkin pie filling), you're likely to find the healthiest option.

VARY IT! Use a full scoop of protein powder if you need more protein to meet your daily target. A full scoop increases your protein intake by about 12–13 grams.

NUTRITION TIP: Pumpkin puree provides beta carotene, which is converted to vitamin A in the body. Vitamin A helps to boost your immune system and supports healthy vision and reproduction.

PER SERVING: *Calories 285 (From Fat 106); Fat 12g (Saturated 1g); Cholesterol 0mg; Sodium 168mg; Carbohydrate 38g (Dietary Fiber 7g); Protein 13g.*

Caramel Coffee Smoothie

PREP TIME: 10 MIN	COOK TIME: NONE	YIELD: 1 SERVING

INGREDIENTS

2 teaspoons instant espresso

1 teaspoon caramel extract

1 tablespoon almond butter

1 scoop chocolate protein powder

1 cup vanilla almond milk

4-5 ice cubes (crushed if necessary)

DIRECTIONS

1 Add instant espresso, caramel extract, almond butter, protein powder, almond milk, and ice to a blender.

2 Blend on high until smooth.

3 Pour into a glass and enjoy.

VARY IT! If you don't have instant espresso, any instant coffee will work. You can also substitute caramel syrup or caramel sauce instead of caramel extract, but it will increase the sugar (and carbohydrate) count.

NUTRITION TIP: This recipe provides about 21 milligrams of caffeine, far less than a cup of coffee, which generally provides about 95mg per cup. You can increase the amount of instant espresso if you want a darker, stronger smoothie. But consider the other caffeinated beverages that you might consume throughout the day. The U.S. Food and Drug Administration recommends no more than 400mg of caffeine per day for healthy adults.

PER SERVING: *Calories 240 (From Fat 117); Fat 13g (Saturated 1g); Cholesterol 0mg; Sodium 259mg; Carbohydrate 13g (Dietary Fiber 3g); Protein 19g.*

Mango Smoothie

PREP TIME: 10 MIN	COOK TIME: NONE	YIELD: 1 SERVING

INGREDIENTS

½ cup frozen mango

½ ripe banana

1 scoop soy protein powder

½ cup vanilla soy milk

½ cup plain soy yogurt

2-3 raspberries (optional)

DIRECTIONS

1 Add mango, banana, protein powder, soy milk, and yogurt to a blender.

2 Blend on high until smooth.

3 Pour into a glass and garnish with raspberries (if desired).

NOTE: The riper the banana, the sweeter your smoothie will be.

VARY IT! Soy milk isn't the only milk alternative that is vegan, but it is usually the one that is highest in protein, depending on the brand. Pea milk (made from pea protein) is another milk alternative that is higher in protein, but it may be harder to find at some markets.

PER SERVING: Calories 329 (From Fat 35); Fat 4g (Saturated 1g); Cholesterol 0mg; Sodium 262mg; Carbohydrate 54g (Dietary Fiber 5g); Protein 23g.

Orange Dreamsicle Smoothie

PREP TIME: 10 MIN	COOK TIME: NONE	YIELD: 1 SERVING

INGREDIENTS

1 orange

½ cup vanilla frozen Greek yogurt

½ cup milk or milk alternative

1 scoop vanilla protein powder

Dollop of whipped cream (optional)

DIRECTIONS

1 Zest the orange to yield about ¼ teaspoon zest and set aside.

2 Peel orange and separate sections.

3 Place orange sections, frozen yogurt, milk, and protein powder into a blender.

4 Blend on high until smooth.

5 Pour into a glass, top with whipped cream, and sprinkle orange zest on top.

VARY IT! If you don't have an orange on hand, use a half cup of orange juice. You can also use orange juice concentrate.

NUTRITION TIP: When shopping for orange juice, look for varieties without added sweeteners. Check the ingredients list for sweeteners such as sugar, honey, grape, or apple juice concentrate.

PER SERVING: *Calories 279 (From Fat 19); Fat 2g (Saturated 0g); Cholesterol 0mg; Sodium 276mg; Carbohydrate 36g (Dietary Fiber 5g); Protein 30g.*

Strawberry Oatmeal Smoothie

PREP TIME: 10 MIN	COOK TIME: NONE	YIELD: 1 SERVING

INGREDIENTS

1 cup strawberries, frozen

¼ cup rolled oats

1 cup oat milk

½ scoop vanilla protein powder

DIRECTIONS

1 Remove stems from strawberries and cut into quarters.

2 Place strawberries, oats, date, oat milk, and protein powder into a blender.

3 Blend on high until smooth.

4 Pour into a glass and enjoy.

PER SERVING: *Calories 291 (From Fat 63); Fat 7g (Saturated 1g); Cholesterol 0mg; Sodium 201mg; Carbohydrate 44g (Dietary Fiber 6g); Protein 13g.*

Chapter **15**

Balanced Breakfasts to Fuel Your Day

RECIPES IN THIS CHAPTER

illing your body with nutritious foods in the morning is a smart way to give yourself the energy you need to fuel your daily activities. And if you balance your macros at the break of day, you'll really stack the deck in your favor.

In this chapter, I share breakfast recipes that provide a healthy balance of nutrients. If you like sweet treats, you'll find some here that can satisfy your cravings while also providing essential protein. If you like a savory meal to start your day, you'll find egg dishes and plant-based options as well. Experiment with different types of foods and even with different portion sizes to see what works best for you.

But do you really need to eat breakfast? Is it better to skip breakfast or eat a big meal first thing in the morning? This chapter also walks you through the breakfast debate so you can decide for yourself.

The Truth about Breakfast

If you are a regular breakfast eater, there's no reason to change your habit. But what if you don't usually eat breakfast? Should you change your habits? And what about all of those studies that were promoted in the media about breakfast and weight loss? If you're trying to lose weight, should you eat right away after waking?

Since 1917, health experts, ads, and promotional campaigns have promoted breakfast as the most important meal of the day. In fact, until just a few years ago, if you considered yourself to be a healthy eater, you didn't go to the gym or head off to work without a hearty morning meal. But views about the health benefits of breakfast have evolved.

It turns out that eating breakfast doesn't always promote weight loss. In fact, several recent studies have debunked the idea that breakfast eaters lose more weight than breakfast skippers. Many factors influence weight loss, and breakfast isn't one that makes a huge difference. What matters most is the overall quantity and quality of your energy (calorie) intake.

REMEMBER

Breakfast eaters should look for foods with fiber, healthy fats, and protein for their morning meal.

While it might be convenient and temporarily enjoyable to grab a sugary baked good (donut, anyone?), that choice might work against you about an hour after you eat it. You're likely to find yourself hungry again and scouring the cabinets or office vending machine for something to eat. A macro-balanced meal, however, takes longer to digest and can help you to feel full and satisfied through the energy slump that so many of us feel around 10 or 11 a.m.

Whether you prefer to enjoy a morning meal or skip breakfast altogether, you won't get an argument here. Your body will tell you if you need to eat. Honor your body's hunger cues and do what works best for you. But don't skip the recipes in this chapter! You can still enjoy breakfast foods for lunch or dinner.

Cottage Cheese Apple Pancakes

PREP TIME: 10 MIN	COOK TIME: 10 MIN	YIELD: 2 SERVINGS *(3 PANCAKES EACH)*

INGREDIENTS

¾ cup small curd, 4 percent cottage cheese

1 egg

¼ cup applesauce

2 tablespoons honey

½ cup flour

¼ teaspoon baking soda

½ teaspoon canola oil

Dash of salt

Maple syrup, butter, or extra applesauce (optional)

DIRECTIONS

1 Put cottage cheese, egg, applesauce, and honey into a food processor or blender and mix until blended.

2 In a medium bowl, combine dry ingredients (flour, baking soda, salt).

3 Add dry ingredients to wet ingredients and mix.

4 Heat a non-stick skillet on medium heat. Add oil to the pan.

5 Pour batter into pan one heaping scoop at a time, making sure to leave space so that the pancakes can spread without running into each other.

6 Wait until the pancakes begin to set. The sides will get dry and small bubbles may form and burst. About 2-3 minutes. Flip with a spatula, and continue cooking until the other side is golden brown, another 2-3 minutes.

7 Plate your pancakes, top with butter, syrup, or applesauce (if desired), and enjoy.

PER SERVING: *Calories 317 (From Fat 67); Fat 7g (Saturated 3g); Cholesterol 118mg; Sodium 591mg; Carbohydrate 47g (Dietary Fiber 1g); Protein 16g.*

Egg and Veggie Breakfast Bake

INGREDIENTS

5 eggs

5 egg whites

⅔ cup low-fat cottage cheese

¾ cup frozen spinach, thawed and well-drained

½ cup sliced mushrooms

1 red bell pepper, diced

½ onion chopped

1 teaspoon garlic powder

½ teaspoon onion powder

½ cup cheddar cheese, shredded

DIRECTIONS

1 Preheat oven to 375. Spray an 8 ½ × 5 ½-inch casserole dish with nonstick cooking spray.

2 In a large bowl, mix together the eggs, egg whites, and cottage cheese until well blended. Add spinach, mushrooms, pepper, onion, and seasonings and stir. Pour into the prepared casserole dish.

3 Bake 40 minutes or until the eggs are set and then sprinkle cheese on top and continue cooking until cheese is melted (about 5 minutes).

4 Remove from oven and allow it to cool slightly before serving.

TIP: This casserole can be made in advance and frozen for later. You can also freeze single servings to reheat in the microwave when you've got a busy morning and need a quick bite.

TIP: If you have it on hand, use about two cups fresh spinach instead of frozen.

NUTRITION TIP: Pair a serving of this egg bake with a half cup of mixed berries for a macro-balanced breakfast.

VARY IT! Use your favorite veggies in this recipe. Do you like a spicy casserole? Add sliced jalapeño. Or experiment with whatever you have in your fridge. Throw in chopped broccoli, asparagus, or even cubed, baked sweet potato.

PER SERVING: *Calories 233 (From Fat 110); Fat 12g (Saturated 5g); Cholesterol 283mg; Sodium 391mg; Carbohydrate 9g (Dietary Fiber 2g); Protein 22g.*

Nutty and Fruity Overnight Oats

PREP TIME: 10 MIN (PLUS OVERNIGHT)	COOK TIME: NONE	YIELD: 2 SERVINGS

INGREDIENTS

½ cup rolled oats

½ cup almond milk

½ cup nonfat Greek yogurt

1 tablespoon chia seeds

½ teaspoon cinnamon

¼ cup sliced almonds

¼ cup fresh or frozen berries

DIRECTIONS

1 In a medium bowl, combine oats, milk, yogurt, chia seeds, and cinnamon. Let the mixture sit for about 5 minutes until the oats start to soften.

2 Divide the mixture into two batches. You'll use one batch to create your first serving and the second batch for the second serving.

3 Layer in a single-serve mason jar (or use a different storage container). First, add half the oat mixture from the first batch, then sprinkle half of the nuts and half of the fruit. Repeat. Use the second batch to create the second serving.

4 Let sit in the refrigerator overnight.

VARY IT! Use your favorite nut instead of almonds. Chopped walnuts work well. Or try pecans, macadamia nuts, or pistachios. If you want to reduce the amount of fat in the recipe, reduce or eliminate the nuts and add a bit more fruit.

NUTRITION TIP: If you want more protein in the morning, add a half scoop of plain or vanilla protein powder to the ingredients in the medium mixing bowl (step 1) to boost your protein intake by 12–13 grams (depending on the protein powder you use).

PER SERVING: *Calories 226 (From Fat 90); Fat 10g (Saturated 1g); Cholesterol 0mg; Sodium 18mg; Carbohydrate 26g (Dietary Fiber 7g); Protein 10g.*

Egg and Avocado Toast

PREP TIME: 10 MIN	COOK TIME: NONE	YIELD: 1 SERVING

INGREDIENTS

1 large slice whole wheat bread

¼ ripe avocado

1 hard-boiled egg, peeled and chopped

1 tablespoon chopped red onion

Salt and pepper to taste

DIRECTIONS

1 Toast the whole wheat bread.

2 Slice avocado, place it on the bread, and mush it down slightly with a fork so it is evenly spread.

3 Top with chopped egg, chopped red onion, salt, and pepper.

VARY IT! The sky's the limit when you're making avocado toast. For instance, if you don't like your eggs hard-boiled, then use a scrambled or fried egg. You can also experiment with toppings that suit your tastes. Try adding hempseeds or chia seeds for a little extra boost of protein. Adding sliced ham or salmon is another great way to add protein. And topping your toast with leafy greens like arugula or spinach gives it extra crunch and volume.

VARY IT! If you avoid gluten, swap out the whole wheat bread for gluten-free bread.

PER SERVING: *Calories 211 (From Fat 102); Fat 11g (Saturated 3g); Cholesterol 212mg; Sodium 219mg; Carbohydrate 18g (Dietary Fiber 3g); Protein 10g.*

Savory Egg White Muffins

PREP TIME: 10 MIN	COOK TIME: 35 MIN	YIELD: 8 MUFFINS

INGREDIENTS

1 tablespoon olive oil

½ cup chopped onion

1 cup red pepper, chopped

1 cup broccoli chopped

½ cup chopped ham

2 cups egg whites

Salt and pepper to taste

DIRECTIONS

1 Preheat oven to 350. Spray a muffin tin with non-stick cooking spray.

2 Heat a non-stick pan over medium heat and add the oil. Sauté onion until softened (about 2-3 minutes). Then add veggies and cook 2-3 minutes more. Add ham and set aside.

3 In a medium bowl, whisk egg whites adding salt and pepper to taste.

4 Spoon the veggie ham mixture into eight muffin cups, dividing it equally. Top with egg mixture.

5 Bake 30 minutes or until the eggs are set.

VARY IT! You can use whatever veggies you have on hand for this recipe. Chopped zucchini, asparagus, tomatoes, or spinach can work well. You can also swap out the meat or eliminate it completely if you prefer. You can add shredded cheese to this recipe to make it heartier.

NUTRITION TIP: Pair an egg white muffin (or two) with whole wheat peanut butter toast for a balanced macro breakfast.

NOTE: Egg muffins freeze well! Make a double batch and freeze them individually so you have them on hand when you need a quick bite. Simply reheat in the microwave and enjoy.

PER SERVING: *Calories 78 (From Fat 24); Fat 3g (Saturated 1g); Cholesterol 8mg; Sodium 126mg; Carbohydrate 4g (Dietary Fiber 1g); Protein 10g.*

Vegan Southwest Tofu Scramble

PREP TIME: 35 MIN   COOK TIME: 10 MIN   YIELD: 2 SERVINGS

INGREDIENTS

8 ounces extra-firm tofu

¼ cup chopped onion

1 tablespoon olive oil

½ red pepper, chopped

½ cup mushrooms

½ cup chopped zucchini

1 teaspoon cumin

1 teaspoon garlic salt

½ cup black beans

1 small jalapeño pepper, sliced

Hot sauce (optional)

DIRECTIONS

1 Use a tofu press to drain the tofu. If you don't have a press, wrap the tofu in a clean dish towel. Place a can or heavy skillet on top so that the liquid drains out. Let it drain for about 30 mins.

2 In a non-stick pan, sauté onion in olive oil over medium heat until softened, about 2–3 minutes. Then add the remaining veggies and cook 2–3 minutes more.

3 In a medium bowl, break the drained tofu into crumbles. Stir in the cumin and garlic salt.

4 Add the tofu mixture and beans to the skillet. Heat until warm.

5 Spoon the scramble onto two plates, top with sliced jalapeño and hot sauce, and enjoy.

NUTRITION TIP: If you are new to tofu, there are great reasons to give it a try. Tofu is an excellent source of complete, plant-based protein. It also provides important minerals, including calcium, manganese, and selenium. Tofu takes on the flavor of whatever it is cooked with, so you can add the seasoning and ingredients that you enjoy to personalize the taste.

VARY IT! If you prefer not to use tofu or if you don't have it on hand, you can make this same recipe with eggs. Use about one cup of eggs or egg whites instead of the tofu. Scramble the eggs in step 3 before adding them to the veggie mix.

VARY IT! Use the veggies that you enjoy for this recipe! Consider adding leafy greens like spinach or kale. Add tomatoes or toss in sliced olives. Top with avocado slices if you have it on hand.

PER SERVING: *Calories 259 (From Fat 117); Fat 13g (Saturated 2g); Cholesterol 0mg; Sodium 1071mg; Carbohydrate 20g (Dietary Fiber 7g); Protein 17g.*

Peanut Butter Yogurt Bowl

| PREP TIME: 5 MIN | COOK TIME: NONE | YIELD: 1 SERVING |

INGREDIENTS

1 cup nonfat Greek yogurt

2 tablespoons creamy peanut butter

1 teaspoon honey

⅛ teaspoon cinnamon

1 tablespoon cacao nibs (optional)

DIRECTIONS

1 Spoon yogurt into bowl.

2 Stir peanut butter vigorously until softened, then blend into yogurt.

3 Drizzle honey on top and sprinkle with cinnamon.

4 Top with cacao nibs (if desired).

VARY IT! Plain yogurt works for this recipe, but you can also try vanilla, chocolate, or banana yogurt, too. And if you prefer a different nut butter, go ahead and swap it out. Try almond butter or cashew butter if you'd like.

NUTRITION TIP: If you want to boost the protein, add a half scoop of chocolate or vanilla protein powder to get an extra 12–13 grams. Stir it into the yogurt before adding your toppings. The protein powder will make your mixture sweeter so you may want to dial back the honey or omit it completely.

NUTRITION TIP: If you want to boost your healthy fat intake top the mixture with nuts or seeds, such as chia seeds, flaxseed, or walnuts.

PER SERVING: *Calories 329 (From Fat 177); Fat 20g (Saturated 6g); Cholesterol 20mg; Sodium 202mg; Carbohydrate 17g (Dietary Fiber 2g); Protein 25g.*

Baked Egg and Sweet Potato

PREP TIME: 10 MIN	COOK TIME: 1 HOUR	YIELD: 2 SERVINGS

INGREDIENTS

1 sweet potato

2 eggs

Salt and pepper to taste

1 cup mixed greens

1 tablespoon olive oil

DIRECTIONS

1 Preheat oven to 400 degrees.

2 Bake sweet potato until soft, about 45–50 minutes.

3 Remove the potato from the oven. Slice in half and place each half on a nonstick baking sheet, skin side down.

4 Using a spoon, scoop out a space in each sweet potato half and crack one egg into each hole, keeping the yoke intact. Sprinkle with salt and pepper.

5 Place the baking sheet back into the oven and bake until the whites are firm and the yokes are set to your preference, about 5–7 minutes.

6 Toss the mixed greens with the olive oil and divide between two plates. Place one half sweet potato on each plate alongside the greens and serve.

NUTRITION TIP: Sweet potatoes provide fiber along with important vitamins and minerals such as vitamin A and vitamin C.

VARY IT! If you'd prefer a recipe with less fat, simply omit the olive oil (which provides about 60 calories of fat per serving). Dress your greens with lemon or balsamic vinegar instead.

PER SERVING: *Calories 327 (From Fat 195); Fat 22g (Saturated 5g); Cholesterol 222mg; Sodium 190mg; Carbohydrate 16g (Dietary Fiber 3g); Protein 20g.*

Oat-ey Protein Waffles

PREP TIME: 10 MIN	COOK TIME: 10 MIN	YIELD: 2 SERVINGS (2-4 WAFFLES)

INGREDIENTS

Cooking spray

2 eggs

1 scoop vanilla protein powder

½ cup plain Greek yogurt

3 tablespoons milk of your choice

½ teaspoon baking soda

½ teaspoon baking powder

¾ cup rolled oats

Fruit or syrup toppings (optional)

DIRECTIONS

1 Preheat waffle iron and spray with cooking spray.

2 Add eggs, protein powder, Greek yogurt, milk, baking soda, baking powder, and rolled oats to a blender and mix until smooth.

3 Spoon batter onto waffle iron and cook until lightly brown.

4 Top with bananas, berries, or maple syrup (if desired) and enjoy.

NOTE: The size of your waffle iron will determine how many waffles this recipe will make. But it should provide two servings.

NOTE: This is a great make-ahead recipe. Double or triple the recipe so you make a big batch of waffles. Then freeze them in single-serve containers. Reheat them in the toaster or microwave when you're ready for a protein-rich meal.

VARY IT!: Get creative with toppings! In addition to fruit or syrup, try your favorite jam, applesauce, or a nut butter.

PER SERVING: *Calories 288 (From Fat 79); Fat 9g (Saturated 3g); Cholesterol 219mg; Sodium 192mg; Carbohydrate 28g (Dietary Fiber 4g); Protein 25g.*

Savory Breakfast Burrito

PREP TIME: 10 MIN	COOK TIME: 10 MIN	YIELD: 2 SERVINGS

INGREDIENTS

2 eggs

½ teaspoon salt

¼ teaspoon chili powder

¼ teaspoon garlic powder

1 teaspoon olive oil

½ cup chopped onion

½ cup chopped red pepper

4 ounces ground turkey or turkey sausage

¼ cup shredded Monterey jack cheese

2 flour tortillas

Salsa or hot sauce (optional)

DIRECTIONS

1 In a small bowl, crack eggs, add seasonings, and whisk vigorously.

2 Add olive oil to a medium skillet and sauté onion and pepper over medium–high heat.

3 Add sausage and continue cooking until the meat is cooked through.

4 Add eggs and scramble the mixture until eggs are cooked to your preference.

5 Divide the cheese between tortillas. Spoon half of the mixture onto each tortilla and fold into a burrito. Top with hot sauce or salsa (if desired) and enjoy.

NUTRITION TIP: The type of turkey that you buy will impact the nutrition facts. Some brands of turkey sausage or ground turkey are almost as high in fat as ground beef. If you prefer a lower-fat breakfast, look for extra lean ground turkey.

VARY IT: Make this a plant-based burrito by using an egg substitute and a vegan cheese alternative. Use soy-based sausage instead of turkey or omit the sausage completely and use black beans instead.

NOTE: This is another great make-ahead meal. Double or triple this recipe and make a batch. Wrap each burrito in foil and store in the freezer until you are ready to eat. Reheat by removing the foil and placing in the microwave covered with a paper towel for about 1 minute.

PER SERVING: *Calories 388 (From Fat 174); Fat 19g (Saturated 7g); Cholesterol 269mg; Sodium 1037mg; Carbohydrate 29g (Dietary Fiber 3g); Protein 24g.*

Chapter 16

Savory Lunches and Dinners

The macro diet is flexible, so you'll have no shortage of options when it comes to lunch and dinner entrees. Regardless of your preferences, you'll be able to enjoy a satisfying meal that helps you reach your nutrient targets.

If you're already comfortable in the kitchen, making macro-balanced meals will be a breeze. You'll find that adding fresh herbs and spices to simple foods can boost flavor without increasing your fat intake too much. And experimenting with different cooking techniques and ingredients can help you to expand your palate so you find new foods to savor and mealtime stays interesting.

If cooking is not your strong suit, that's okay! The recipes in this chapter are great for cooks at every level. (But if you only trust yourself with an Easy-Bake Oven, you may want to phone a friend for help.) Spicy Slow Cooker Chili, for example, is nearly impossible to mess up, and it's a meal that you can enjoy in a variety of different ways. The Super Easy Three Bean Salad requires no cooking at all, and if you want to impress your friends or family, make beginner-friendly shrimp and veggie kebobs on the grill.

In this chapter, I walk you through the basics of cooking macro-friendly meals, help you create delicious no-cook meals, and share some of my favorite lunch and dinner recipes.

Cooking Macro-Friendly Meals

As you learn to make lunch and dinner on your own, just remember that you want to build meals that include a variety of ingredients to enhance flavor and increase your intake of all three macros.

Following this three-step process in order will help you reach your targets.

1. **Choose a protein** like fish or lean meat, or a plant-based protein like tofu. Remember that a typical serving size is 100 grams or about 3.5 ounces. But that isn't necessarily the correct portion for you. (A *"serving size"* is the amount listed on the Nutrition Facts label and *"portion"* is the actual amount you consume. See Chapter 6 for details.) Adjust your portion as needed so that you hit your protein goal.

2. **Next, add healthy carbs.** After you've got your protein figured out, think about adding veggies and/or a starch. Choose your favorite greens, a seasonal vegetable, or whatever you have on hand. If the veggie that you choose is a little higher in starch, you might not want to add another carb. A sweet potato, for example, is technically a vegetable, but it provides plenty of starch (along with fiber and naturally occurring sugar), so you wouldn't necessarily need to add another starchy food to your meal. But if you choose sauteed spinach as your veggie, you could supplement it with a serving of brown rice, farro, or whatever starchy carb you prefer.

3. **Finally, let fat take care of itself.** In most cases, you'll hit your fat target without intentionally adding fat to your plate. Marinades, salad dressings, and other toppings, for instance, often provide fat. If you sauté veggies in avocado oil or brush your fish with olive oil before you broil it, you may get enough fat to hit that target. And remember that most dairy products provide some fat as well.

Making Meals at Home without Cooking

If you experiment in the kitchen and decide that cooking is not for you, you still have good ways to maintain a macro diet.

Many meal delivery programs accommodate macro-trackers. On many of their websites, for example, you'll see the nutritional breakdown of each meal before you choose your selections, so you can select the options that work best for you. But if budget is a concern, these delivery services may not be your best bet as they tend to be a bit pricey.

If meal delivery is not an option for you, take some time to check out healthy prepared foods at the grocery store. Consider these tips as you explore:

TIP

>> **Look in the meat department for prepared entrees.** Often, you'll find lean turkey burgers, seasoned seafood, marinated poultry, and other options that are ready to grill or bake.

>> **Find veggies that are already washed and prepped in the produce department or freezer aisles.** All you have to do is heat them in the microwave.

>> **Salad kits are another option as a side dish or a full meal, although sometimes the toppings and dressings are not very nutritious.**

   You can always drizzle olive oil on your salad instead of using the dressing that is provided. Also, you can supplement these salads by adding protein (canned tuna, beans, shredded chicken, nuts, or seeds), and you can bulk up the salad by adding more greens or veggies.

>> **The deli section is also likely to have salads and other entrees available.** Grain and bean salads are great choices. You might also find egg salad or seafood salads here. Unfortunately, however, you're not always able to see nutritional information for these foods, so it can be hard to determine the amount of fat, sodium, or added sugar.

An old-school rule of thumb is to shop the perimeter of the grocery store to find the freshest, healthiest choices. Often the freezer section and the center aisles are full of foods that are more heavily processed and contain ingredients that you might not want. As consumers have become more nutrition-savvy, food manufacturers have responded by delivering higher-quality packaged foods, but that old-school rule still holds true to a great extent.

REMEMBER

Always read the nutrition labels so you know what you're getting as you make your selections.

Hearty Greek Salad

PREP TIME: 35 MIN	COOK TIME: NONE	YIELD: 6 SERVINGS

INGREDIENTS

3 large skinless, boneless chicken breasts (about 5–6 ounces), grilled

2 tablespoons olive oil

For the dressing:

¼ cup extra virgin olive oil

3 tablespoons red wine vinegar

2 cloves garlic, minced

1½ teaspoons dried oregano

½ teaspoon salt

¼ teaspoon pepper

For the salad:

3 cups chopped romaine lettuce

1 cucumber, peeled, sliced and quartered

1 cup cherry tomatoes, halved

¾ cup kalamata olives, pitted

¼ cup artichoke hearts, quartered

8 ounces feta cheese, crumbled

DIRECTIONS

1 Preheat your grill to medium high heat. Brush the grates with oil.

2 Place the chicken breasts on the grill, leaving space between each one so that heat can circulate. Close the grill lid.

3 Grill for about 6 to 8 minutes per side. Cooking time will vary based on the thickness of the breasts. When the chicken looks done, check the internal temperature in the thickest part of the breast and be sure it registers at least 165 degrees.

4 Remove chicken from the grill and let it rest while you assemble other ingredients. If you cook the chicken in advance, refrigerate the chicken until you are ready to add it to the salad.

5 Whisk together all of the dressing ingredients in a medium bowl and set aside.

6 In a large salad bowl, combine all of the salad ingredients except the chicken; then drizzle the dressing on top.

7 Lightly toss the salad and divide among six plates.

8 Slice the chicken breasts and top each salad with half a breast.

9 Salt and pepper to taste and enjoy.

TIP: If you're not going to eat all six servings at once, you can prep the dressing, the chicken, and all of the veggies in advance, but keep them in separate air-tight containers in the refrigerator. That way, all of the veggies will stay crisp. Then combine the salad ingredients, toss with the dressing, and top with chicken breast just before serving.

NUTRITION TIP: If you are watching your sodium intake, look for low-sodium feta or try rinsing your feta before using it in the recipe to reduce the salt a bit. Choose artichoke hearts that are not marinated in oil, as they usually also contain quite a bit of salt. You can also eliminate the olives, to reduce the sodium even further.

VARY IT! The ingredients listed here are typical for a Greek salad, but you can experiment with other additions. You might try adding red pepper, grilled eggplant, or even green beans. No chicken breast on hand? Try grilled salmon or tuna to keep the salad protein-rich.

TIP: In a hurry? If you are short on time, you can use pre-cooked chicken that you find in some grocery stores' butcher departments or freezer sections. Try to avoid processed deli meat as it may have higher levels of sodium, and deli meats, in general, have been linked to an increased risk of heart disease, cancer, and diabetes.

PER SERVING: *Calories 253 (From Fat 202); Fat 22g (Saturated 8g); Cholesterol 41mg; Sodium 687mg; Carbohydrate 5g (Dietary Fiber 1g); Protein 9g.*

Ground Turkey Sweet Potato Skillet

PREP TIME: 10 MIN	COOK TIME: 30 MIN	YIELD: 4 SERVINGS

INGREDIENTS

2 tablespoons olive oil, divided

1 large onion, diced

1 pound 85 percent lean ground turkey

3 cups sweet potato, diced (about 2 to 3 sweet potatoes)

1 yellow pepper, diced

1 teaspoon garlic powder

1 teaspoon paprika

1 teaspoon cumin

½ teaspoon chili powder

½ cup shredded pepper jack cheese

DIRECTIONS

1 Preheat oven to 400 degrees.

2 In a large oven–safe skillet, heat one tablespoon olive oil over medium heat and sauté the onion until translucent, about 2 to 3 minutes.

3 Add the turkey to the skillet. Cook until lightly browned, about 5 to 7 minutes.

4 Add another tablespoon of olive oil; add the sweet potato and continue cooking until it begins to soften; add diced yellow pepper and cook until peppers begin to soften.

5 Add seasonings to the skillet and stir. Cover the mixture and let cook for about 10 to 12 minutes until the sweet potatoes are tender. Stir the mixture occasionally and add a tablespoon or two of water if the skillet becomes dry.

6 When the veggies are soft, top with pepper jack cheese and put the skillet (uncovered) into the oven until the cheese is melted.

7 Let cool slightly and serve warm.

TIP: This skillet dish reheats well. Make a big batch and store in air-tight, single-serve containers either in the refrigerator (for 3 to 4 days) or in the freezer.

VARY IT! If you are watching your fat or calorie intake, choose extra lean ground turkey for this recipe. But you'll need to add a little extra liquid (use water or chicken stock) during the cooking process.

NUTRITION TIP: Sweet potatoes are a great source of healthy carbs. You'll get almost 4 grams of fiber in each sweet potato that you consume, along with protein, vitamin A, vitamin C, and potassium.

PER SERVING: *Calories 386 (From Fat 200); Fat 22g (Saturated 6g); Cholesterol 97mg; Sodium 201mg; Carbohydrate 21g (Dietary Fiber 3g); Protein 27g.*

Simple Egg Salad

PREP TIME: 20 MIN	COOK TIME: NONE	YIELD: 4 SERVINGS

INGREDIENTS

8 hard-boiled eggs

2 stalks celery, chopped

½ cup onion, chopped

½ cup dill pickles, chopped

½ cup plain, nonfat Greek yogurt

2 teaspoons yellow mustard

Salt and pepper to taste

DIRECTIONS

1 Peel and chop the hard-boiled eggs.

2 In a medium bowl, combine the eggs, celery, onion, and dill pickles.

3 In a separate bowl, mix together the Greek yogurt and mustard to make the dressing.

4 Add the dressing to the egg mixture and stir gently until combined.

5 Salt and pepper to taste.

TIP: Egg salad is so versatile! Enjoy it alone or slather it on whole wheat bread to make an open-faced egg salad sandwich. Scoop it into a pita if you'd like or drop a dollop onto a cucumber slice and enjoy it as a quick snack. Keep egg salad refrigerated for up to four days.

NUTRITION TIP: Egg whites are a good source of leucine, an essential amino acid that has been studied for its potential muscle-building and weight-loss properties.

VARY IT! Use Dijon mustard if you prefer it over yellow mustard. And if you don't have any mustard on hand, just add a tablespoon of mustard powder and a dash of salt to the Greek yogurt.

PER SERVING: Calories 189 (From Fat 101); Fat 11g (Saturated 4g); Cholesterol 425mg; Sodium 489mg; Carbohydrate 6g (Dietary Fiber 1g); Protein 15g.

Curried Lentil Soup

PREP TIME: 10 MIN	COOK TIME: 60 MIN	YIELD: 8 SERVINGS

INGREDIENTS

2 tablespoons olive oil

1 medium onion, chopped

4 carrots, peeled and chopped

3 garlic cloves, minced

4 teaspoons curry powder

½ teaspoon cumin

1 16-ounce package dried lentils, rinsed

8 cups chicken stock

Salt and pepper to taste

Plain Greek yogurt for topping (optional)

DIRECTIONS

1 In a large pot, heat the olive oil on medium heat and sauté the onion until translucent.

2 Add the carrots and cook until the carrots begin to soften, about 5 minutes.

3 Add the garlic and the spices. Stir until the vegetables are well coated.

4 Add the lentils and continue to stir until the lentils are lightly toasted — about 3 minutes.

5 Add chicken stock and bring to a boil. Reduce the heat and simmer until the lentils are soft, about 1 hour.

6 Season with salt and pepper.

7 Serve in a bowl, topped with a dollop of plain Greek yogurt (if desired).

TIP: This soup is best when it is made in advance and allowed to cool before reheating. Make it in the afternoon for a hearty warm dinner or make a big pot to keep in the fridge so that you can enjoy it for several days.

NOTE: You can use green or brown lentils for this recipe. Brown lentils will get a bit softer than green ones and have an "earthier" flavor.

NUTRITION TIP: Lentils are a versatile and nutritious source of plant-based protein. They also provide folate and fiber. You can buy lentil soup to get these health benefits, but store-bought soups are often high in sodium.

VARY IT! Use vegetable stock if you prefer a vegan or vegetarian option. Keep in mind, however, that not all vegetable stocks are vegan. Check the label to make sure that there are no animal ingredients (such as gelatin). Then use a non-dairy Greek yogurt to top the soup.

PER SERVING: *Calories 294 (From Fat 49); Fat 5g (Saturated 1g); Cholesterol 0mg; Sodium 791mg; Carbohydrate 41g (Dietary Fiber 19g); Protein 20g.*

Easy Chicken Taco Casserole

INGREDIENTS

1 pound skinless, boneless chicken breast

1½ cups cooked brown rice

1 can black beans, rinsed and drained

2 red peppers, diced

1 cup corn (frozen or canned)

½ cup sliced black olives

1 8-ounce container plain Greek yogurt

1 packet taco seasoning

1 cup shredded Monterey jack cheese

DIRECTIONS

1 Fill a large pot with water. Add the chicken breast and bring to a boil. Reduce heat and simmer until chicken is cooked through, about 15 to 20 minutes. The internal temperature at the thickest part should measure at least 165 degrees.

2 Allow the chicken to cool slightly and then shred the chicken using two forks.

3 Preheat oven to 375 degrees. Spray a 9 by 13-inch baking pan with non-stick cooking spray.

4 In a large bowl, combine the chicken, rice, beans, peppers, corn, olives, yogurt, and seasoning mix.

5 Spoon the mixture into the baking pan, cover with foil, and bake for 30 minutes. Remove the foil, sprinkle the cheese on top, and bake for another 5 minutes until the cheese is melted.

VARY IT! Add more veggies if you'd like to bulk up this recipe. Chopped zucchini or tomatoes work well in taco casserole.

NUTRITION TIP: Seasoning mixes (like taco seasoning) can be high in sodium. If you are watching your salt intake, omit the seasoning packet. Use a 2-tablespoon mixture of cumin, garlic powder, and chili pepper to get the same Tex-Mex taste. Use about 1 teaspoon each for a spicy blend or dial back the chili pepper and add a bit more cumin and garlic powder if you prefer a milder seasoning.

PER SERVING: Calories 257 (From Fat 68); Fat 8g (Saturated 4g); Cholesterol 29mg; Sodium 297mg; Carbohydrate 30g (Dietary Fiber 7g); Protein 18g.

Cool Couscous and Lentil Salad

PREP TIME: 15 MIN	COOK TIME: 10 MIN	YIELD: 4 SERVINGS

INGREDIENTS

For the salad:

1 cup Moroccan couscous

1 teaspoon olive oil

4½ cups water

1 cup green lentils, rinsed

1 cup cherry tomatoes, halved

1 cup cucumbers, sliced and quartered

¼ cup red onion, chopped

¼ cup crumbled feta

For the dressing:

3 tablespoons olive oil

2 tablespoons red wine vinegar

1 tablespoon lemon juice

1 teaspoon honey

1 clove garlic, minced

DIRECTIONS

1 In a medium pot, add three cups of water and the lentils. Bring to a boil. Reduce heat to a simmer, cover, and cook until lentils are tender, about 20 minutes. Remove from heat and drain any excess water. Let cool.

2 In a medium pot, bring the remaining water (1 ½ cups), olive oil, and couscous to a boil. Keeping the pot covered, remove it from the heat and let sit for 5 minutes. Fluff the couscous with a fork and let it cool.

3 Make the dressing. Add all of the dressing ingredients to a small bowl and whisk until combined.

4 Combine the lentils, veggies, feta, and couscous in a medium bowl. Drizzle the dressing on top and toss until coated. Divide among four plates.

NOTE: If you don't have the dressing ingredients on hand, or if you are in a hurry, use a bottle of vinaigrette instead. You can also just use a few tablespoons of olive oil in a pinch.

VARY IT! Experiment with different types of couscous. Pearl couscous (sometimes called Israeli couscous) is an option if you prefer a "meatier" grain. You can also substitute white or brown rice, but couscous is lower in calories and carbs. Experiment with the type of lentil you use, but green lentils tend to hold their shape the best.

PER SERVING: *Calories 478 (From Fat 127); Fat 14g (Saturated 3g); Cholesterol 8mg; Sodium 116mg; Carbohydrate 68g (Dietary Fiber 18g); Protein 20g.*

Spicy Slow Cooker Chili

PREP TIME: 5 MIN   COOK TIME: 6 HOURS   YIELD: 8 SERVINGS

INGREDIENTS

1 tablespoon olive oil

1 medium onion chopped

3 garlic cloves, minced

1½ pounds lean ground beef

2 16-ounce cans dark red kidney beans, drained and rinsed

1 28-ounce can crushed tomatoes

2 4-ounce cans diced green chiles

1 cup beef broth

2 tablespoons chili powder

½ teaspoon cayenne pepper

Salt and pepper to taste

Shredded cheese, sour cream, sliced green onion (optional)

DIRECTIONS

1 In a large skillet, heat the olive oil on medium heat and sauté the onion and garlic until translucent.

2 Add the beef and cook until browned, breaking it up as it cooks.

3 Transfer the beef to your slow cooker. Add the beans, tomatoes, green chiles, broth, and spices. Stir the mixture to combine.

4 Cook on high for 6 hours.

5 Season with salt and pepper.

6 Serve in a bowl with shredded cheese, sour cream, or sliced green onion (if desired).

NUTRITION TIP: Use your protein of choice for this recipe. Many people prefer ground turkey instead of beef when they make chili simply because it has less fat. You might also consider ground bison, which is usually leaner than beef but has a gamier flavor.

VARY IT! You can make this recipe your own in many ways! Use black beans instead of red kidney beans. You can also use canned chili beans that already have spices added to them. If you prefer a less spicy chili, omit the green chilis and the cayenne pepper. You can even toss in some sliced green olives!

NOTE: Enjoy this chili "Cincinnati style" if you want to boost your carb intake. Spoon the chili onto a small serving of cooked plain spaghetti and top with shredded cheese, onions, and/or soda crackers for a hearty meal.

PER SERVING: *Calories 337 (From Fat 137); Fat 15g (Saturated 5g); Cholesterol 58mg; Sodium 707mg; Carbohydrate 27g (Dietary Fiber 8g); Protein 24g.*

Thai Chicken Lettuce Wraps

INGREDIENTS

For the filling:

1 tablespoon olive oil

1 pound ground chicken

½ yellow onion, diced

½ red pepper diced

½ green pepper diced

1 can water chestnuts, diced

For the sauce:

3 tablespoons soy sauce

1 tablespoon sesame oil

1 tablespoon rice vinegar

2 teaspoons minced fresh ginger

1 teaspoon sugar

2 tablespoons hoisin sauce

For the wraps:

1 head Boston bibb lettuce

¼ cup green onions, sliced

DIRECTIONS

1 Add oil to a large skillet and brown the ground chicken over medium heat.

2 Add the onion, peppers, and water chestnuts. Sauté until the onion is translucent and the vegetables are starting to soften.

3 While the veggies are cooking, whisk together the sauce ingredients in a small bowl.

4 Pour the sauce into the skillet and stir until the meat and veggies are well coated.

5 Separate at least four whole lettuce leaves from the head, keeping the leaves intact. Place one large scoop of the chicken mixture into each leaf. Top with green onions, and enjoy.

VARY IT! Make this a plant-based meal by using firm tofu, tempeh, or jack fruit instead of chicken. Be sure to press the water out of the tofu before cooking (see package instructions). Then cook it just like you'd cook the chicken, making sure to break it into crumbles as it heats up.

TIP: If you are watching your salt intake, choose low-sodium soy sauce, but keep in mind that even the low-sodium variety may contain almost 600mg of sodium per serving. You can also use tamari if you are gluten-free; even though tamari is made without (or with very little) wheat, it still may contain some gluten. Check the label to be sure.

PER SERVING: *Calories 310 (From Fat 149); Fat 17g (Saturated 4g); Cholesterol 98mg; Sodium 985mg; Carbohydrate 18g (Dietary Fiber 4g); Protein 23g.*

Honey Mustard Glazed Salmon

PREP TIME: 10 MIN	COOK TIME: 15 MIN	YIELD: 4 SERVINGS

INGREDIENTS

2 cloves garlic, minced

2 tablespoons whole-grain mustard

1 tablespoon honey

1 tablespoon soy sauce

Four 4 to 6 ounce salmon filets

DIRECTIONS

1 Preheat oven to 400 degrees.

2 Make the glaze by combining all ingredients except salmon in a small bowl and whisking together.

3 Pat the salmon filets dry. Place on a baking sheet lined with parchment paper, skin side down. Brush glaze over salmon so that each filet is evenly coated.

4 Place the salmon in the oven and bake until it is cooked to your preference, about 15 minutes.

TIP: Enjoy this salmon with a serving of brown rice and a side of green veggies, like green beans, asparagus, or wilted spinach, for a macro-balanced meal.

NUTRITION TIP: Salmon is not only a good source of protein, but it also provides omega-3 fatty acids, which can reduce your risk of "heart failure, coronary heart disease, cardiac arrest and the most common type of stroke (ischemic)," according to the American Heart Association.

PER SERVING: *Calories 181 (From Fat 61); Fat 7g (Saturated 1g); Cholesterol 59mg; Sodium 278mg; Carbohydrate 6g (Dietary Fiber 0g); Protein 25g.*

Crunchy Chicken Hummus Wrap

PREP TIME: 10 MIN	COOK TIME: NONE	YIELD: 1 SERVING

INGREDIENTS

2 tablespoons hummus

1 large spinach and herb tortilla

4 ounces grilled, sliced chicken breast

Sliced radishes

Shredded carrots

Sliced cucumber

Green leaf lettuce

DIRECTIONS

1 Spread the hummus on a flat tortilla.

2 Layer grilled chicken on top of the hummus.

3 Add veggies according to your preference.

VARY IT! If you can't find spinach tortillas, use large flour tortillas instead. You can also use whatever veggies you have on hand. Toss in tomatoes, shredded jicama, cabbage, or avocado to make this meal heartier!

TIP: Grill a few chicken breasts in advance so you have them on hand to make sandwiches for a few days.

PER SERVING: *Calories 461 (From Fat 109); Fat 12g (Saturated 3g); Cholesterol 96mg; Sodium 606mg; Carbohydrate 42g (Dietary Fiber 4g); Protein 43g.*

Healthy Tuna Poke Bowl

PREP TIME: 10 MIN	COOK TIME: NONE	YIELD: 2 SERVINGS

INGREDIENTS

For the bowl:

1 cup cooked rice

¼ pound sushi-grade tuna, cubed

½ ripe avocado cubed

½ cup soybeans, shelled and cooked

½ cup radishes, thinly sliced

½ cup shredded carrots

¼ cup scallions, sliced

1 teaspoon black sesame seeds

For the dressing:

2 tablespoons light mayonnaise

2 teaspoons sriracha sauce

DIRECTIONS

1 Divide the ingredients so that you can assemble the food into two single-serve bowls. Add the rice first to the bottom of the bowl. Place the tuna on top of the rice in the middle and then scoop the avocado, soybeans, radishes, and carrots into separate "piles" on top of and around the tuna. Sprinkle the scallions and sesame seeds on top. Repeat for the second bowl.

2 Whisk together the mayo and sriracha sauce. Drizzle over bowl ingredients.

VARY IT! You don't have to use sushi-grade tuna for this recipe; you can use canned tuna (or even cubed chicken or tofu) instead. But the flavor won't be the same. Sushi-grade tuna has a flavor that is more meaty and less fishy. But keep in mind that sushi-grade fish is only good refrigerated for 1 to 2 days, so if you want to make this ahead of time, sushi grade may not be the best option.

PER SERVING: *Calories 332 (From Fat 122); Fat 14g (Saturated 2g); Cholesterol 31mg; Sodium 150mg; Carbohydrate 33g (Dietary Fiber 6g); Protein 21g.*

Baked Pork Chops with Mashed Cauliflower

PREP TIME: 10 MIN	COOK TIME: 30 MIN	YIELD: 4 SERVINGS

INGREDIENTS

For the pork chops:

Four 5 to 6 ounce bone-in pork chops, about 1 inch thick

2 tablespoons brown sugar

1 teaspoon paprika

½ teaspoon garlic salt

½ teaspoon oregano

For the mashed cauliflower:

1 large head cauliflower

2 tablespoons cream cheese

2 tablespoons butter

Salt and pepper

2 tablespoons chives, chopped

DIRECTIONS

1 Preheat the oven to 375 degrees.

2 Pat pork chops dry and set aside.

3 In a small bowl, combine the brown sugar, paprika, garlic salt, and oregano. Rub the mixture on the pork chops.

4 Place the pork chops on a baking sheet lined with parchment paper. Place the baking sheet in the oven and bake the chops for about 25 minutes or until the internal temperature reaches 145 degrees.

5 While the pork chops are cooking, remove any leaves from the cauliflower and break it into large chunks (florets). Place the cauliflower in a steaming basket or colander and put the basket into a large saucepan. Add about one inch of water to the bottom of the saucepan, cover, and place it on high heat. Steam until the cauliflower is tender, about 10 to 12 minutes.

6 Put the butter and cream cheese into a food processor. Add the tender cauliflower florets and process until creamy. Add salt and pepper to taste.

7 When the pork reaches 145 degrees, remove it from the oven and let the chops rest on a plate covered with foil for 5 minutes.

8 Place one pork chop and a scoop of mashed cauliflower on each of four plates. Sprinkle chives on the cauliflower and serve.

NOTE: Some people enjoy their pork slightly pink; check the meat juices to determine whether it is cooked to their liking. Usually, if the juices run clear or slightly pink, the meat is cooked. However, the U.S. Department of Agriculture (USDA) advises that you use a meat thermometer to check the temperature of pork. If you remove the pork from the heat at 145 degrees, it will continue to cook while it rests so that the meat is safe to eat and still juicy and tender after 3 to 5 minutes.

NUTRITION TIP: Mashed cauliflower is a great substitute for mashed potatoes. You get the same creamy taste and texture, but cauliflower also provides fiber, vitamin C, vitamin B6, magnesium, calcium, iron, and phosphorus.

VARY IT! This meal is hearty on its own, but it also pairs well with sautéed spinach or steamed green beans if you would like to add another veggie.

PER SERVING: *Calories 325 (From Fat 127); Fat 14g (Saturated 7g); Cholesterol 121mg; Sodium 456mg; Carbohydrate 15g (Dietary Fiber 4g); Protein 36g.*

Grilled Shrimp Kebobs

PREP TIME: 35 MIN	COOK TIME: 10 MIN	YIELD: 4 SERVINGS

INGREDIENTS

2 pounds raw, peeled, deveined shrimp

¼ cup olive oil

2 tablespoons lemon juice

2 garlic cloves, minced

1 teaspoon paprika

½ teaspoon coriander

¼ teaspoon red pepper flakes

DIRECTIONS

1 Pat the shrimp dry. Preheat the grill on high heat.

2 Add the remaining ingredients to a large bowl and stir to combine.

3 Add the shrimp to the bowl and toss until coated. Let the shrimp marinate in the refrigerator for 30 minutes.

4 Thread shrimp onto stainless steel skewers, alternating direction and making sure that the shrimp barely touch.

5 Reduce the grill temperature to low. Grease the cooking grates and place the shrimp skewers on the grill. Close the grill cover and cook for 2 to 3 minutes per side until the shrimp are no longer translucent.

NOTE: Round out your meal by adding a few veggie skewers to the grill as well. Thread mushroom caps, yellow or green peppers, cherry tomatoes, zucchini, or onions onto a skewer and grill alongside the shrimp. Serve just with the shrimp or on top of basmati rice if you prefer.

NUTRITION TIP: Shrimp is a great source of complete protein. It is low in fat, easy to cook, and an excellent source of vitamin B12 — a nutrient that is important for healthy blood and nerve cells.

PER SERVING: *Calories 362 (From Fat 157); Fat 17g (Saturated 3g); Cholesterol 345mg; Sodium 336mg; Carbohydrate 3g (Dietary Fiber 0g); Protein 46g.*

Super Easy Three Bean Salad

PREP TIME: 10 MIN	COOK TIME: 10 MIN	YIELD: 4 SERVINGS

INGREDIENTS

For the salad:

One 15-ounce can red kidney beans

One 15-ounce can black beans

One 15-ounce can cannellini beans

½ cup chopped red onion

½ cup chopped celery

⅓ cup chopped parsley

For the dressing:

¼ cup olive oil

¼ cup red wine vinegar

1 teaspoon honey

1 teaspoon Dijon mustard

Salt and pepper to taste

DIRECTIONS

1 Drain and rinse the beans. Add them to a large bowl with the onion, celery, and parsley.

2 In a separate bowl, combine the dressing ingredients and whisk until combined.

3 Drizzle the dressing over the bean mixture and toss until the beans and veggies are well coated.

VARY IT! Want to make this meal heartier and more nutritious? Add green beans! Simply steam a batch of beans, cut them into 1-inch segments, and toss them in. Also, don't worry if you don't have the beans mentioned here. Use whatever you have on hand. Try pinto beans, wax beans, navy beans, or even lima beans if you'd like.

NUTRITION TIP: Beans are a great way to add protein and fiber to almost any meal. So, it is smart to always have a few cans on hand. But canned beans might provide added sodium. Check the ingredients list if you are concerned about your salt intake. Then always rinse beans before using them in recipes. You can also cook dry beans at home. Follow package instructions for best results, but most beans cook to a tender texture in about 40 to 45 minutes (even without soaking!).

PER SERVING: *Calories 451 (From Fat 142); Fat 16g (Saturated 2g); Cholesterol 0mg; Sodium 693mg; Carbohydrate 50g (Dietary Fiber 20g); Protein 19g.*

Italian Meatball Casserole

PREP TIME: 10 MIN	COOK TIME: 10 MIN	YIELD: 6 SERVINGS

INGREDIENTS

For the meatballs:

1 pound extra lean ground beef (or ground turkey)

½ cup chopped onion

¼ cup breadcrumbs

¼ cup parmesan cheese

1 egg

1 tablespoon Italian seasoning

For the casserole:

One 16-ounce box whole wheat rigatoni pasta

One 24-ounce jar marinara sauce

4 ounces fresh mozzarella, sliced

Fresh basil (optional)

DIRECTIONS

1 Preheat the oven to 350 degrees.

2 Make the meatballs by adding all the meatball ingredients to a large bowl and mixing with your hands until well combined.

3 Shape the mixture into 1-inch meatballs and place them on a baking sheet (about 30 meatballs).

4 Bake the meatballs for about 25 to 30 minutes until fully cooked through and evenly browned.

5 While the meatballs are baking, prepare the pasta. Begin by boiling a large pot of water. Add the pasta and bring to a boil again. Reduce the heat slightly and cook until the pasta is al dente (firm with a slight chew), about 10 minutes.

6 Drain the pasta and transfer to a large oven-safe casserole dish.

7 Add the meatballs to the casserole dish and top with marinara sauce. Arrange mozzarella slices on top and put the casserole back into the 350-degree oven.

8 Bake for another 15 minutes or until the cheese is melted and the casserole is hot.

9 Garnish with fresh basil and serve.

NUTRITION TIP: Your favorite marinara or spaghetti sauce may contain high levels of sodium and even added sugar. Read the Nutrition Facts label or the ingredient list to be sure you know what you're getting. You can also use plain tomato sauce for this recipe if you prefer.

PER SERVING: *Calories 596 (From Fat 130); Fat 14g (Saturated 6g); Cholesterol 103mg; Sodium 748mg; Carbohydrate 78g (Dietary Fiber 6g); Protein 36g.*

snacks are good for your diet

» Whipping up protein-rich sweets and treats

Chapter **17**

Desserts, Snacks, and Treats

RECIPES IN THIS CHAPTER

- ↻ **Protein Brownie-in-a-Cup**
- ↻ **No-Bake Pumpkin Protein Balls**
- ↻ **Sweet Pepper Nut Poppers**
- ↻ **Healthier Mock Deviled Eggs**
- ↻ **Spicy Roasted Chickpeas**
- ↻ **Protein Peanut Butter Cups**
- ↻ **Nutty Homemade Protein Bars**
- ↻ **Oven-Baked Kale Chips**

f your favorite meal of the day is dessert, then you will love this chapter. When you're tracking your macros, you can still enjoy sweet treats and other snacks.

REMEMBER

In fact, if sweets and snacks make you happy, then you *should* include them in your diet. You're not likely to stick to a plan that leaves you feeling deprived. So, it is important to include these foods in your meal plan if you enjoy them to make your eating plan more sustainable.

And not only can snacks and sweets make your eating plan easier to maintain, they can also help you to reach your macro targets. Usually, snack foods are full of carbs and fat. But you can also boost your protein intake in many ways when you indulge in treats. In this chapter, you'll find recipes that use protein-powder, nuts, nut butter, and other ingredients so that each food has a balance of all three macros.

Protein Brownie-in-a-Cup

PREP TIME: 10 MIN	COOK TIME: 10 MIN	YIELD: 1 SERVING

INGREDIENTS

1 scoop chocolate protein powder

½ container Greek yogurt (5.3-ounce cup)

1½ tablespoons water

2 tablespoons peanut butter powder

1 teaspoon baking powder

1 tablespoon peanut butter

DIRECTIONS

1 Spray the inside of a mug with non-stick cooking spray.

2 In a small bowl, mix all of the ingredients except the peanut butter. Stir until combined.

3 Pour brownie batter into a mug. Microwave on high for 40 seconds.

4 Stir. Microwave again for 20 to 30 seconds.

5 Remove from microwave, top with peanut butter, and enjoy.

PER SERVING: *Calories 378 (From Fat 131); Fat 15g (Saturated 4g); Cholesterol 20mg; Sodium 406mg; Carbohydrate 22g (Dietary Fiber 4g); Protein 45g.*

No-Bake Pumpkin Protein Balls

PREP TIME: 10 MIN	COOLING TIME: 30 MIN	YIELD: 25–30 BALLS

INGREDIENTS

1½ cups rolled oats

2 scoops vanilla protein powder

⅔ cup almond butter

½ cup pumpkin puree

¼ cup maple syrup

1 teaspoon pumpkin pie spice

¼ cup mini chocolate chips

Dash of salt

DIRECTIONS

1 Combine all ingredients in a medium bowl and mix well.

2 Refrigerate for an hour or until the dough thickens.

3 Using a teaspoon, scoop out dough and form it into balls.

4 Refrigerate for 30 minutes before serving.

5 Store in the refrigerator for up to 5 days.

PER SERVING: *Calories 72 (From Fat 36); Fat 4g (Saturated 1g); Cholesterol 0mg; Sodium 53mg; Carbohydrate 7g (Dietary Fiber 1g); Protein 3g.*

BUYING PRE-MADE TREATS AND SNACKS

If you don't have time to spend in the kitchen, don't worry. More and more companies are making desserts and snacks with the macro-counter in mind. Check out Greek yogurt bars or protein-rich frozen treats in the freezer section of your local grocery store. In the snack section, you'll find fiber-rich popcorn, crunchy veggie-based chips, and protein bars to choose from.

Keep in mind that these convenience foods generally don't provide as many micronutrients as other foods (like fruits, vegetables, lean meats, and grains), and they are often high in calories. If you're following the macro diet to lose weight, consuming these foods in moderation may be the smartest approach.

Sweet Pepper Nut Poppers

INGREDIENTS

1 pound bag of mini sweet peppers (about 12 peppers)

48 Marcona almonds

6 ounces Manchego cheese, sliced thin

DIRECTIONS

1 Preheat oven to 400 degrees.

2 Halve each pepper and lay on a baking sheet lined with parchment.

3 Into each pepper half, place two almonds and a sprinkle of cheese.

4 Bake for about 15 minutes until almonds are soft and cheese is melted.

PER SERVING: *Calories 322 (From Fat 189); Fat 21g (Saturated 11g); Cholesterol 45mg; Sodium 189mg; Carbohydrate 17g (Dietary Fiber 6g); Protein 18g.*

VARY IT! Pepper poppers are a versatile food. They make a great snack and an even better appetizer to serve at parties. If you want more protein, sauté some lean ground turkey with Italian seasonings and add a spoonful to each pepper.

NOTE: Marcona almonds are softer and more moist than regular almonds, so you'll get a better texture if you use them (rather than regular almonds).

Healthier Mock Deviled Eggs

PREP TIME: 10 MIN	COOK TIME: NONE	YIELD: 6 SERVINGS

INGREDIENTS

6 large hard-boiled eggs

½ cup prepared hummus

Chopped chives (optional)

DIRECTIONS

1 Peel hard-boiled eggs. Slice each egg in half lengthwise. Remove the yolks.

2 Place a generous half tablespoon of hummus into each egg half.

3 Top with chives and serve.

NUTRITION TIP: There is nothing wrong with traditional deviled eggs or the yolks of hard-boiled eggs. The benefit of this recipe is that it has a better macro balance. While hard-boiled eggs and traditional deviled eggs provide fat and protein, they provide little carbohydrate. By replacing the yolk with hummus, you give your body nutritious carbohydrates, including fiber.

PER SERVING: Calories 113 (From Fat 63); Fat 7g (Saturated 2g); Cholesterol 211mg; Sodium 189mg; Carbohydrate 5g (Dietary Fiber 1g); Protein 7g.

Spicy Roasted Chickpeas

PREP TIME: 5 MIN	COOK TIME: 25 MIN	YIELD: 6 SERVINGS

INGREDIENTS

Two 15-ounce cans of chickpeas (garbanzo beans)

1 teaspoon ground cumin

1 teaspoon smoked paprika

1 teaspoon garlic powder

1 teaspoon chili powder

2 tablespoons olive oil

DIRECTIONS

1 Preheat oven to 400 degrees.

2 Drain and rinse chickpeas. Pat dry.

3 In a small bowl, mix together seasonings and set aside.

4 In a medium bowl, toss the chickpeas with the olive oil. Add spice mixture and toss until evenly coated.

5 Spread in a single layer on a baking sheet. Bake for 30 minutes, shaking the pan every 10 minutes or so.

6 Remove from the oven and serve hot or allow to cool and store in an airtight container for up to 2 weeks.

PER SERVING: *Calories 235 (From Fat 72); Fat 8g (Saturated 1g); Cholesterol 0mg; Sodium 300mg; Carbohydrate 32g (Dietary Fiber 9g); Protein 10g.*

Protein Peanut Butter Cups

INGREDIENTS

1½ cup dark chocolate chips

1 tablespoon coconut oil

3 tablespoons vanilla protein powder

⅓ cup peanut butter

DIRECTIONS

1 Place paper liners into eight wells of a muffin tray.

2 Place the chocolate chips and coconut oil into a microwave-safe glass bowl. Place it in the microwave and cook on high for up to 2 minutes. Check the mixture every 30 seconds or so to see whether it is melted. Stir until the mixture is combined.

3 Pour half the chocolate mixture into the six wells of the muffin tin, dividing equally. Set the other half of the melted chocolate aside. Pick up the tin and tilt it in different directions so that the chocolate creeps up the sides of each liner. Place the tin in the freezer for about 10 minutes until the chocolate hardens.

4 Add the peanut butter to a small bowl and add one tablespoon of protein powder. Stir vigorously to combine. Repeat with the other two tablespoons of protein powder. Make sure the mixture is not drippy. If it is, add more protein powder.

5 Refrigerate the mixture for 30 minutes.

6 Use a small spoon to scoop out the peanut mixture and roll it into eight small balls. Place one ball on top of each chocolate well in the muffin tin.

7 Use the remaining chocolate mixture to top each peanut butter ball. Place the muffin tin back into the freezer for another 10 minutes.

NOTE: Store the peanut butter cups in the freezer until you are ready to enjoy them.

VARY IT! Use whatever nut butter you prefer. Try almond butter, cashew butter, or macadamia nut butter. Also, if you don't have coconut oil on hand, you can use butter, but coconut oil gives a better texture.

PER SERVING: *Calories 241 (From Fat 150); Fat 17g (Saturated 8g); Cholesterol 0mg; Sodium 75mg; Carbohydrate 23g (Dietary Fiber 3g); Protein 6g.*

Nutty Homemade Protein Bars

INGREDIENTS

1 4-ounce package of pitted Medjool dates (about 6 dates)

1¾ cups rolled oats

1 cup peanut butter

⅓ cup honey

1 cup vanilla protein powder

½ cup ground flaxseed

½ cup coconut flakes

DIRECTIONS

1 Place dates in a food processor and process until they form a ball.

2 Mix together the remaining ingredients, except the coconut flakes, in a separate bowl. Add the mix to the food processor and blend until combined. Add a teaspoon or so of water if the mix is too dry.

3 Press the mixture onto a baking sheet lined with parchment paper. Use a larger sheet if you want thinner bars or a smaller sheet if you want thicker bars. The mixture doesn't need to cover the entire sheet. Sprinkle coconut on top.

4 Place the sheet in the refrigerator. Cool for about one hour. Remove from the fridge and cut into individual squares. Wrap each in parchment and store in the refrigerator.

PER SERVING: *Calories 339 (From Fat 166); Fat 18g (Saturated 7g); Cholesterol 0mg; Sodium 165mg; Carbohydrate 35g (Dietary Fiber 6g); Protein 14g.*

Oven-Baked Kale Chips

PREP TIME: 5 MIN	COOK TIME: 25 MIN	YIELD: 4 SERVINGS

INGREDIENTS

1 pound curly kale (about one large bunch), rinsed and dried

1 tablespoon olive oil

1 teaspoon sea salt

DIRECTIONS

1 Preheat oven to 300 degrees.

2 Remove the stems from each kale leaf. Break the remaining kale leaves into bite-sized pieces.

3 In a large bowl, toss the leaves with the olive oil and salt.

4 Spread onto a large baking sheet lined with parchment and place the baking sheet in the oven.

5 Bake for 20 to 25 minutes or until the chips are crispy.

NUTRITION TIP: Kale has gotten a bad rap over the years, but it is highly nutritious. It provides a small amount of protein, along with vitamins C, A, and K.

VARY IT! Experiment with different flavor combinations. Use cumin and garlic salt for Mexican-style chips, try cheddar powder or nutritional yeast for a cheesy kale chip, or try Italian seasoning for a zesty flavor.

PER SERVING: *Calories 87 (From Fat 38); Fat 4g (Saturated 1g); Cholesterol 0mg; Sodium 517mg; Carbohydrate 11g (Dietary Fiber 2g); Protein 4g.*

Chapter **18**

Make-Ahead Meal Prep Ideas

A sk anyone who has successfully used macro tracking to meet health or fitness goals, and they will tell you that meal prep is the key to success.

TIP Preparing meals in advance ensures that you have nutritious foods ready to go when you need them. And since your nutrition tracking has been done in advance, you can ensure that they are prepared in a way that helps you meet whatever macro goals you've set for yourself.

In this chapter, I share some recipes that can be prepared ahead of time, making mealtime and macro tracking a breeze. These meals can be prepared as indicated in each recipe. But take some time to read the variations and notes after each one. You can also adjust the portion sizes for starchy foods (like grains and pasta) or veggies to meet your needs. You can modify these recipes in dozens of ways so that they give you the balance of nutrients that you are looking for and the flavors that you desire.

Meal Preparation and Storage Tips

Eager to jump right into your first meal prep adventure? No problem! Here are a few essential tips that can help get you started. If you'd rather start by discovering the differences between different storage containers, tools to have on hand, and tips for reheating, venture over to Chapter 8, where I explain everything you need to know about weekly meal prep in detail.

>> **Tailor recipes to meet your needs.** You can use the nutrient data provided, but if you modify the recipe, you'll want to recalculate the numbers. Remember to weigh foods raw rather than cooked when gathering nutrient data for the most accurate results.

>> **Store foods in airtight containers that are microwave-safe.** Glass containers work well, but there are also plastic options available that can go in the microwave. Just be sure to read labels before buying. You can even look for containers with separate compartments.

>> **Consider your microwave's settings.** Reheating times can vary based on the meal and your microwave. Usually, it'll take 1 to 3 minutes to reheat a meal. But keep in mind that foods with more fat cook more quickly than foods with more water. Try microwaving each meal for 1 minute and then stir and reheat in 20-minute intervals until your food is warm.

>> **Reheat food without Tupperware lids.** It is usually not a good idea to keep container lids on when reheating food. Instead, use a damp paper towel. It will prevent the food from spraying over the inside of the microwave and will help to keep your food from drying out.

>> **Use the oven.** If you prefer not to use a microwave, you can reheat meals in the oven instead. Use an oven-safe container and heat for about 10 to 20 minutes at 350 degrees. Stove-top reheating also works for some meals.

Almost all of the recipes included in this chapter are for four meals. That is because the meals only stay fresh for about four days in the refrigerator.

TIP

A few of the recipes do well in the freezer (especially Spaghetti and Turkey Meatballs). For those recipes, feel free to double or triple the recipe and keep the extra meals in the freezer.

Spaghetti and Turkey Meatballs

PREP TIME: 30 MIN	COOK TIME: 20 MIN	YIELD: 8 MEALS

INGREDIENTS

For the meatballs:

2 pounds Italian-seasoned lean ground turkey

2 cups Italian breadcrumbs

1 large onion, diced

½ cup milk

2 large eggs

4 cloves garlic, minced

1 teaspoon salt

1 teaspoon pepper

For the pasta:

1 16-ounce package whole grain spaghetti

2 24-ounce jars low sodium spaghetti sauce

DIRECTIONS

1 Preheat the oven to 400 degrees.

2 In a large bowl, combine the ground turkey, breadcrumbs, egg, milk, garlic, salt, and pepper. Use your hands to mix well.

3 Roll the meat mixture into about 32 balls, approximately 1.5 to 2 inches in diameter.

4 Place on a non-stick (or greased) baking sheet and bake for about 20 minutes or until cooked through.

5 While the meatballs are cooking, boil the pasta in a large pot according to package instructions.

6 Drain the pasta and set aside.

7 When the meatballs are cooked to an internal temperature of 160 degrees, divide the pasta between eight single-serve containers. Top each serving of pasta with four meatballs and then top with about ½ cup of sauce. Refrigerate the meals that you plan to eat in the next four days and freeze the rest.

NOTE: If you can't find Italian-seasoned ground turkey, you can use a tablespoon or two of Italian seasoning. Add it during step 2.

NOTE: When reheating pasta, it is always helpful to add just a bit of water or extra sauce to keep it from getting dry. Also remember, to cover with a damp paper towel so that the meat and the pasta stay moist and flavorful.

NUTRITION TIP: Serve your meal with a mixed green salad or steamed veggies to boost your veggie intake. If you like spinach, you can also just stir a handful or two right into your meal to increase your intake of leafy greens.

PER SERVING: *Calories 672 (From Fat 4163); Fat 18g (Saturated 5g); Cholesterol 142mg; Sodium 981mg; Carbohydrate 92g (Dietary Fiber 6g); Protein 39g.*

Meatloaf with Sweet Potato Mash and Green Beans

PREP TIME: 30 MIN	COOKING TIME: 1 HOUR	YIELD: 4 MEALS

INGREDIENTS

For the meatloaf:

1 pound lean ground beef

1 small onion, chopped

1 large egg

1 clove garlic, minced

⅓ cup Italian breadcrumbs

3 tablespoons milk

½ teaspoon salt

½ teaspoon pepper

For the potatoes:

1½ pounds sweet potatoes
(about 3 to 4 potatoes)

1 tablespoon butter

2 tablespoons maple syrup

2 tablespoons milk

Dash of salt

For the green beans:

1 pound fresh green beans, trimmed

DIRECTIONS

1 Preheat the oven to 400 degrees. Spray a non-stick baking sheet with non-stick spray (or line it with parchment) and set aside.

2 When the oven is preheated, place the sweet potatoes in the oven directly on the rack.

3 Place the meatloaf ingredients in a medium bowl and use clean hands to combine well.

4 Form four small loaves with the meat mixture and place each one on the prepared baking sheet, leaving space between each loaf. Place the sheet in the oven with the potatoes and bake for 30 to 40 minutes until each loaf is cooked through to an internal temperature of 160 degrees.

5 When the potatoes are soft (about one hour in the oven) remove the skin and put the de-skinned potatoes into a medium bowl with the butter, maple syrup, milk, and salt. Use a handheld mixer to whip the potatoes until fluffy. Set aside.

6 Prep the beans. Heat a medium saucepan with about an inch of water to boiling. Add the beans and cook until the beans are bright green (but not soft), about 1 to 2 minutes. Remove from heat and rinse in cool water to stop the cooking process.

7 Assemble the meals in single-serve containers. Place one meatloaf, a big scoop of potatoes, and green beans into each container. Cover and refrigerate for up to four days.

NOTE: You can double this recipe for eight meals so that you have four to freeze. However, some people don't like the texture of mashed sweet potatoes when they are thawed and reheated. My suggestion is to double the meatloaf recipe, then after packing four meals, package the remaining loaves individually and freeze. Then when you're ready to create four new meals, thaw the loaves and make a new batch of potatoes and veggies.

NOTE: No fresh green beans? Use frozen! They are equally nutritious and don't need to be precooked. Simply add a cup to each meal container.

PER SERVING: *Calories 464 (From Fat 152); Fat 17g (Saturated 7g); Cholesterol 136mg; Sodium 670mg; Carbohydrate 49g (Dietary Fiber 7g); Protein 31g.*

Baked Chicken Thighs with Rice and Peas

PREP TIME: 10 MIN	COOK TIME: 30 MIN	YIELD: 4 MEALS

INGREDIENTS

For the chicken:

1 teaspoon garlic powder

1 teaspoon onion powder

½ teaspoon paprika

½ teaspoon oregano

½ teaspoon thyme

½ teaspoon rosemary

4 chicken thighs, bone-in, skin-on

1 tablespoon olive oil

Salt and pepper to taste

For the rice:

1 cup long-grain rice

½ teaspoon salt

2 cups water

For the peas:

2 cups frozen peas

DIRECTIONS

1 Preheat oven to 400 degrees. Spray a baking sheet with non-stick spray.

2 Combine seasonings in a large mixing bowl.

3 Drizzle olive oil onto chicken thighs. Add the thighs to the mixing bowl and toss until well coated with the spice mixture.

4 Place the seasoned chicken thighs on the baking sheet and place the sheet in the oven. Bake for 30 to 35 minutes or until the internal temperature reaches 170 degrees. Set chicken aside.

5 While the chicken thighs are cooking, prepare the rice. Add salt to 2 cups of water in a medium saucepan and bring to a boil. Add the rice, cover, and reduce the heat to a low simmer for about 20 minutes. Remove from heat and fluff with a fork.

6 Prepare single-serve meals. Place one chicken thigh, ½ cup rice, and ½ cup frozen peas into each container. Refrigerate for up to four days.

VARY IT! Boost your whole grain intake by using brown rice instead of white rice. You can also use another grain of choice, such as quinoa, farro, barley, or couscous.

VARY IT! Choose your frozen veggie of choice. Use frozen broccoli, green beans, or mixed veggies if you prefer.

TIP: If you like spicier food, double the spice mixture for a more flavorful dish.

NUTRITION TIP: If you're looking for a leaner meal, use skinless, boneless chicken breasts instead of chicken thighs. Watch the serving size, though. Many chicken breasts are 7 to 8 ounces or more. So, each breast can provide more than one serving depending on your macro targets and desired portion size. After cooking and before assembling meals, slice the chicken breast into 1-inch slices to make reheating easier.

PER SERVING: *Calories 371 (From Fat 114); Fat 13g (Saturated 3g); Cholesterol 48mg; Sodium 409mg; Carbohydrate 46g (Dietary Fiber 4g); Protein 17g.*

Roasted Veggie Grain Bowl

PREP TIME: 10 MIN	COOK TIME: 30 MIN	YIELD: 4 MEALS

INGREDIENTS

For the grains:

½ cup dry quinoa, rinsed

1 cup water or stock

For the veggies:

2 bell peppers, chopped and deseeded

1 medium zucchini, sliced

1 yellow squash, sliced

½ cauliflower head, chopped

1 can chickpeas, drained and rinsed

2 tablespoons olive oil

1 teaspoon dried oregano

¼ teaspoon garlic powder

Salt and pepper to taste

1 cup prepared hummus (optional)

DIRECTIONS

1 Preheat oven to 400 degrees.

2 In a large bowl, toss the vegetables and chickpeas with olive oil, oregano, and garlic powder until well coated.

3 Spread veggie mixture evenly on a baking sheet, sprinkle with salt and pepper, and place in oven. Bake for about 20 minutes. Toss the veggies once; then return to the oven for another 10 minutes or until the vegetables are cooked to your desired texture.

4 While the vegetables are roasting, cook the quinoa. Combine the water and quinoa in a medium saucepan and bring to a boil. Cover, reduce the heat, and simmer for about 15 minutes. Remove the saucepan from the heat (keeping it covered) and let it stand for 5 minutes. Fluff with a fork.

5 When quinoa is cooked and veggies are ready, prepare single-serve containers. Divide quinoa evenly among four containers, then top each with one-fourth of the vegetables. Place a dollop of hummus in the corner of each meal kit (or in a small individual container).

6 Refrigerate containers for up to four days.

NOTE: You can enjoy this meal chilled (right out of the fridge), at room temperature, or warmed up. If you choose to reheat the veggie bowls, be sure that the hummus is separated from the veggies until after the reheating is complete.

NOTE: If you've never cooked quinoa before and you're not sure how to tell when it is done, look for a white "tail" that appears around each grain. This tells you that the grain has softened and is ready to remove from the heat.

NUTRITION TIP: If you'd like to bulk up this recipe, add nutrient-rich seeds. Pumpkin seeds, sunflower seeds, or chia seeds add crunch, fiber, and healthy fat to this meal.

VARY IT! If you prefer more flavorful quinoa, cook it in chicken or vegetable stock. Just be aware that it will increase the sodium level of your meal. If you want the flavor without high sodium, look for low-sodium stock or use a blend of half water and half stock.

VARY IT! This is a basic recipe that can be adapted to fit any grain and vegetable combination. Choose farro, couscous, brown rice, white rice, or a combination of grains. Then get creative with veggies and simply use what you have on hand. Add mushrooms, cherry tomatoes, red onion, or broccoli. The hummus is optional, and you can even experiment with different sauces. Peanut sauce works, or even a hot sauce.

PER SERVING: *Calories 308 (From Fat 98); Fat 11g (Saturated 1g); Cholesterol 0mg; Sodium 213mg; Carbohydrate 43g (Dietary Fiber 11g); Protein 12g.*

Spicy Cauliflower and Black Bean Taco Bowl

PREP TIME: 30 MIN	COOK TIME: 30 MIN	YIELD: 4 MEALS

INGREDIENTS

For the cauliflower:

1 teaspoon smoked paprika

1 teaspoon cumin

1 teaspoon garlic powder

1 teaspoon chili powder

1 head of cauliflower, separated into 1-inch florets

2 tablespoons olive oil

For the rice:

1 cup long-grain white rice, uncooked

2 cups water

Dash of salt

For the taco bowl:

1 15-ounce can of black beans, rinsed and drained

1 cup canned or frozen corn

1 bunch green onions (whites and light green sections only) sliced

1 jalapeno pepper, deseeded and sliced

Salsa or hot sauce (optional)

DIRECTIONS

1 Preheat oven to 400 degrees. Cover a baking sheet with parchment and set aside.

2 Place cauliflower florets in a large bowl with the oil and toss to coat.

3 In a medium bowl, combine the spices. Add the spices to the cauliflower bowl and toss to coat the cauliflower with the spice mixture.

4 Spread the cauliflower evenly on the baking sheet and place in the oven. Bake for 20 to 30 minutes, until the florets are lightly brown and crispy. Remove from oven and set aside.

5 While the cauliflower is roasting, prepare the rice. Bring water to a boil in a medium saucepan. Add the salt and rice, cover, and reduce the heat to a simmer. Cook for 18 to 20 minutes (without removing the cover). Remove from the heat and let sit for 5 minutes. Fluff with a fork.

6 When the cauliflower and rice are cooked, begin to prepare the individual bowls. Divide the rice between four separate meal containers. On each one, place one-quarter of the cauliflower and one-quarter of the beans. Add a quarter cup of corn; then top with green onion and jalapeno slices.

7 Refrigerate for up to four days. Enjoy this meal cold, at room temperature, or reheated. Add hot sauce or salsa (if desired) when you're ready to eat.

NOTE: Some people don't like the texture of roasted cauliflower. If you prefer it more tender, parboil the cauliflower for 1 to 2 minutes and drain before tossing with the spices and roasting.

NUTRITION TIP: Boost your calcium intake if you'd like. Add a dollop of sour cream, Greek yogurt, or a quarter cup of cheese.

VARY IT! Add more protein to this meal if you need more of that macro to reach your targets. Use shredded chicken or pulled pork. Either roast and shred the meat yourself, or if you're short on time, check your local market. Many stores carry shredded meats to use in recipes.

VARY IT! If you'd like to add protein but you want to keep this recipe plant-based, use tofu instead. You'll want to use firm tofu that is well-drained (see package instructions). Cube the tofu and toss it in a teaspoon of olive oil and bit of the spice mixture that you used for the cauliflower. Then bake it (at 400 degrees) or pan-fry it until it is brown and crispy.

PER SERVING: *Calories 376 (From Fat 69); Fat 8g (Saturated 1g); Cholesterol 0mg; Sodium 195mg; Carbohydrate 65g (Dietary Fiber 10g); Protein 13g.*

Cajun Shrimp and Soba Noodles

PREP TIME: 15 MIN	FREEZE TIME: 20 MIN	YIELD: 4 MEALS

INGREDIENTS

For the noodles:

1 8–9 ounce package of soba noodles

2 cups water

1 teaspoon Cajun seasoning (see **"Cajun Spice Mix"** recipe that follows)

For the shrimp:

2 cups shrimp, raw, deveined, tails off

1 tablespoon Cajun seasoning

2 tablespoons olive oil

1 small onion, chopped

2 bell peppers (red, green or orange), chopped

1 cup spiralized or shredded carrot

2 tablespoons sesame seeds, toasted (optional)

Soy sauce (optional)

DIRECTIONS

1 Prepare the soba noodles. Bring water to a boil over high heat. Add the noodles, cover, and lower the heat to a simmer. Cook until noodles are just tender, about 6 to 8 minutes. Drain the noodles and rinse in cool water to stop the cooking process. Toss one teaspoon of Cajun spice blend to season the noodles. Set aside.

2 Pat shrimp dry. Place in a medium bowl and toss them with the one tablespoon of Cajun seasoning.

3 Place a medium skillet over medium heat. Add the oil. When the oil is hot, add the onion and sauté until the onions are tender.

4 Add peppers to the pan and sauté for about 5 minutes.

5 Add the shrimp to the pan. Shake the pan occasionally so the shrimp cook evenly on all sides. Continue to cook until the shrimp are done (they are pink in color) and the peppers have softened. Remove from heat and toss in the carrots. Stir the mixture and set aside.

6 Prepare the individual meals. Divide the soba noodles into four single-serve containers. Top each container with one-quarter of the shrimp and veggie mixture. Sprinkle sesame seeds on top.

7 Refrigerate for up to four days. Enjoy chilled or reheated. Drizzle soy sauce on top for extra flavor.

NOTE: Soba noodles are a type of Japanese pasta made from buckwheat flour. If you can't find them in the pasta aisle at your local market, check the International Foods aisle. They may be on the shelves near other Japanese foods.

NOTE: Be sure not to overcook soba noodles. They get soggy quickly.

VARY IT! Want more flavor? Instead of boiling the soba noodles in water, cook them in dashi, an umami-rich Japanese soup stock. You'll find it in Asian markets or at some grocery stores in the International Foods aisle.

VARY IT! If you can't find soba noodles (or prefer not to use them), use whole-wheat spaghetti instead.

NOTE: If you don't have Cajun seasoning on hand, you can make your own.

Cajun Spice Mix

2 teaspoons paprika

2 teaspoons garlic powder

1 teaspoon onion powder

1 teaspoon dried oregano

1 teaspoon cayenne pepper

1 teaspoon salt

½ teaspoon black pepper

¼ teaspoon red chili flakes

Combine all of the ingredients and store in an airtight container away from heat and light.

PER SERVING: *Calories 473 (From Fat 91); Fat 10g (Saturated 2g); Cholesterol 237mg; Sodium 981mg; Carbohydrate 56g (Dietary Fiber 3g); Protein 41g.*

Twice Baked Potato Burgers

PREP TIME: 20 MIN	COOKING TIME: 60 MIN	YIELD: 4 MEALS (2 SKINS EACH)

INGREDIENTS

4 large Idaho potatoes, scrubbed clean

2 tablespoons olive oil, separated

Kosher salt

1 medium onion, chopped

1 10-ounce bag fresh spinach

1 pound extra lean ground beef

1 tablespoon butter

2 tablespoons milk

1 teaspoon salt

½ cup shredded cheddar cheese

DIRECTIONS

1 Preheat the oven to 400 degrees.

2 Using one tablespoon of olive oil, brush each potato with oil until lightly coated. Sprinkle each potato with kosher salt and place them in the oven. Bake for about 45 minutes until the skins are crispy and the insides are tender.

3 Place a large skillet over medium heat and add the other tablespoon of olive oil. Add the onion and sauté until tender. Add the spinach and cook until softened. Add the ground beef and continue cooking until the meat is cooked through and no longer pink, about 5 to 7 minutes.

4 Prepare the potatoes. Slice each potato in half, preserving the skins. Scoop out the middle potato and add it to a mixing bowl with the butter and milk. Mix with a handheld mixer until fluffy.

5 Assemble the potatoes. Divide the meat and spinach mixture between each of the eight potato skins. Top each one with mashed potatoes and sprinkle cheese on top. Place the assembled potato skins on a baking sheet. Place the baking sheet back in the oven and heat until the cheese is melted, about 5 minutes.

6 Place the skins in an air-tight container and refrigerate for up to four days. Reheat in the oven or the microwave when you're ready to eat.

NUTRITION TIP: Decrease the fat if you prefer by using extra lean ground turkey instead of beef.

NUTRITION TIP: Even though this recipe includes veggies, you can up your intake by pairing this meal with a mixed green salad or steamed veggies.

NOTE: This is a great recipe to make in batches and freeze.

PER SERVING: *Calories 631 (From Fat 187); Fat 21g (Saturated 8g); Cholesterol 93mg; Sodium 869mg; Carbohydrate 73g (Dietary Fiber 9g); Protein 38g.*

Thai Chicken and Rice Bowl

TIME: 10 MIN	COOK TIME: 30 MIN	YIELD: 4 MEALS

INGREDIENTS

For the chicken:

½ tablespoon chili oil

1 pound ground chicken

½ cup dark brown sugar

¼ cup bottled hot sauce of your choice

2 tablespoons rice wine vinegar

1 teaspoon ground ginger

For the rice:

1 cup long-grain white rice

2 cups water

Dash of salt

For the bowls:

2 cups shredded carrots

1 bunch green onions (whites and light green sections), sliced

DIRECTIONS

1 Heat a large non-stick skillet over medium heat. Add the chili oil and chicken. Cook the chicken, breaking it into crumbles as it cooks.

2 Add the brown sugar, hot sauce, rice wine vinegar, and ginger to a bowl and mix. Then add the sauce to the chicken and mix until the chicken is cooked through and the spice mixture is incorporated. Set aside.

3 Make the rice. Add salt to 2 cups of water in a medium saucepan and bring to a boil. Add the rice, cover, and reduce the heat to a low simmer for about 20 minutes. Remove from heat and fluff with a fork.

4 Assemble the bowls. Divide the rice between four single-serve containers and top each with a quarter of the spicy chicken mixture. Add a scoop of shredded carrots and top with green onions.

5 Store in the refrigerator for up to four days and reheat at mealtime.

NOTE: You can keep the carrots and green onions in snack-sized baggies if you prefer for those veggies to stay crunchy when you enjoy this meal. That way they stay cool and crunchy when you reheat the chicken and rice.

NOTE: Use lean ground turkey if ground chicken isn't available.

PER SERVING: *Calories 445 (From Fat 103); Fat 11g (Saturated 3g); Cholesterol 96mg; Sodium 250mg; Carbohydrate 62g (Dietary Fiber 3g); Protein 24g.*

6

The Part of Tens

Gain cooking confidence and banish food boredom with chef-inspired methods for making mouth-watering dishes.

Discover smart and savvy market hacks that help you make healthy choices when you shop (and do it in less time!).

Choose from delicious, sweet, savory, and nutritious portable snacks for those on the go.

Chapter **19**

Ten Ways to Add Flavor to Protein (without Added Fat or Carbs!)

etting enough protein is a primary goal for many macro trackers — especially those who pair the macro diet with a workout program. Studies and other data collected by government agencies show that most Americans get enough protein to meet their basic needs, but studies suggest that Americans consume more protein (and more animal protein) than other countries around the world. Still, meeting basic protein needs is different than meeting protein needs for a specific training goal (such as weight loss or building muscle).

TECHNICAL STUFF

Protein requirements in the U.S. are similar to those in Canada, Norway, and other countries throughout Europe.

When you increase your intake to support a training program, you may have to put special effort into getting high-quality protein in your diet. And you may want to do so without adding too many grams of fat and carbohydrate so your macros stay balanced.

To keep your diet interesting and enjoyable, you'll want to explore various ways to cook different types of *traditional* protein, including red meat, poultry, pork, seafood, and tofu. Sure, you can add store-bought sauces and dressings to give flavor to your meal, but often, these contain added sugar and fat.

If you prefer not to add fat and carbs, this chapter gives you some techniques to explore different flavors and make your macro-balanced meals more delicious.

Vary Your Prep Methods

The cooking technique that you use will contribute to the taste and texture of your food. Usually, cooking methods are divided into two categories:

>> **Dry heat** involves heating the protein without moisture. For instance, grilling, broiling, and roasting use dry heat. Dry heat is best used with tender cuts of meat, such as those that have some marbling (fat) or are from the loin area of the animal.

>> **Moist heat** involves cooking meat with liquids, such as braising, poaching, or stewing. Moist heat is often used with tougher cuts of meat (like a tough cut of beef) because the lower temperature and the moisture help to break down connective tissue.

Within each of these categories are different methods you might use to prepare meat, poultry, or seafood. Some of these can be used to prepare tofu as well.

>> **Braising** is a moist method in which your protein is wrapped in foil or is in a covered container. A small amount of liquid is added (such as water or broth) to create steam that cooks the meat or seafood.

>> **Grilling** uses dry radiant heat and is the perfect method if you want that chargrilled taste. Steak, poultry, and many types of seafood, such as salmon, tuna, and swordfish, work well on the grill. You can also grill firm tofu.

>> **Roasting** is slower than other cooking methods, but it is great if you have a flavorful piece of protein and want to draw out lots of flavor over time. Roasting is a dry method and takes place in your oven, usually at temperatures in the 300 to 400 degree range. Roasting works well if you have a whole chicken, a turkey, or a large cut of meat, such as roast beef.

>> **Sautéing** is a moist method. You cook your protein in a small amount of fat or oil on your stovetop. It is generally considered to be a lower-fat method of cooking as compared to methods like frying, where your meat (or tofu) is immersed in fat. Many cooks sauté vegetables to bring out their flavor, but you can also sauté certain types of seafood, like shrimp or scallops.

>> **Stir-frying** is a moist method that uses oil, like sautéing but you'll use higher heat with this method. It is best if you can stir-fry in a wok (a bowl-shaped frying pan) so that you can stir and toss thin slices of protein and veggies to cook them without having the food sit in oil. Stir-frying works well with thin cuts of beef, poultry, shellfish, and tofu.

TIP

You can learn more about these different techniques by taking a cooking class or checking out classes online or on television. You may even want to explore other techniques that go beyond these basic methods.

The way you cook meat, seafood, or tofu can add as much to the taste of the protein as a marinade or spice blend. If you have the time, it's worth it to learn a variety of methods.

Make a Marinade

A marinade is basically a bath for your meat or protein. It is a liquid solution that adds flavor and can help to tenderize your meat, poultry, seafood, or tofu.

Usually, a marinade includes three components: an acid (like vinegar, wine, or citrus); an oil, such as olive oil; and some seasoning, such as herbs or spices. But you don't have to include all three elements if you don't want to.

If you want to omit the oil, you can. Although keep in mind that using oil in a marinade won't add substantial fat to your meal.

If you want to make a fat-free marinade, try using lemon, lime, or orange juice as the base. Then add herbs like thyme, rosemary, and garlic. Marinate your protein for a few hours prior to cooking.

Create a Zesty Spice Blend

You have endless options when you experiment with different spices and spice blends. The most basic combinations will include salt, pepper, and perhaps onion or garlic salt. But you can also add cayenne pepper for extra heat or cumin for a warm, earthy, and pungent taste.

Premade spice blends are also a great option. You might start with a basic spice blend like Old Bay (easily found in the spice aisle of most supermarkets) for poultry or seafood. But you can also find a wide array of blends in the spice aisle that include spices like curry, coriander, and chili powder.

TIP

Keep in mind that some spice blends contain a lot of sodium. So if you are watching your salt intake, be sure to read labels.

Savor Smoky Flavors

If you like foods with a smoky flavor, find different types of paprika to use to flavor your meat, pork, poultry, or tofu.

Paprika is a deep red spice made from dried peppers. It has a bit of heat to it, and some people say that it also adds a bit of sweetness to foods.

Your local grocery store will have basic paprika in the spice aisle. But you can choose many artisan spices as well, including smoked paprika that gives meat that salty, tangy flavor that most people describe as smoky. If you like it, look into other types of paprika, such as hot paprika (made from hot chili peppers), Hungarian paprika, or Spanish Paprika (called Pimentón).

Grow (or Buy) Herbs

Fresh herbs like basil, rosemary, cilantro, mint, tarragon, or chives add freshness and flavor to grilled or baked pork, chicken, seafood, and tofu. Visit the produce section of your local market to find seasonal herbs, especially in the summer.

TIP

If you want to save a few bucks, grow your own herbs at home — even if you don't have a green thumb! Visit a garden store (or online vendor) and get a basic kit to grow herbs in your kitchen. Keep them in a window and watch them grow. Then snip them off and use them to add flavor to eggs, salads, and veggies dishes.

You can also use dried herbs. They last longer and are easier to use than the fresh variety. No chopping is needed!

To use herbs on your protein, make a rub by combining herbs with garlic and a small amount of olive oil (optional) to bind the mix together. Then slather your meat, chicken, or tofu and throw it on the grill, into the oven, or into a sauté pan.

Boost the Umami with Soy Sauce or Tamari

If you like foods that have a rich, savory taste, then you'll want to use flavor techniques that boost umami, the fifth basic taste (in addition to sweet, salty, sour, and bitter).

Umami is often described as "complex" or "meaty" and somewhat similar to "salty."

Two flavoring agents that bring out the umami in your protein are soy sauce and tamari. Most people have soy sauce in their condiment shelf in the refrigerator.

TIP

You can marinate your protein in soy sauce or just sprinkle some on after cooking. Use low-sodium soy sauce if you're watching your salt intake.

Tamari is similar to soy sauce but less common. It is also made from fermented soybeans (like soy sauce) but it contains no wheat (soy sauce does contain wheat). So, if you follow a gluten-free diet, choose tamari to make sure you don't get any hidden gluten.

Make the Most of Mustard

Have you visited the condiment aisle of your grocery store lately? The mustard selection has exploded. If you're used to simply grabbing the bright yellow bottle and moving on, you might want to linger for a minute and check out the other options.

You now have endless choices when it comes to different types of mustard and all of them can be slathered on different types of protein to add flavor.

You might try brushing chicken or seafood with a mix of Dijon mustard, honey or brown sugar, and a touch of vinegar for a tangy glaze. Spicy brown mustard, whole grain mustard, and hot mustard might be used as a dipping sauce for your favorite meat or seafood. You'll even find artisan mustards made with ingredients like cherries or raspberries.

Brush on a Balsamic Glaze

Balsamic vinegar is a dark, concentrated style of vinegar that originated in Italy but can be found in any supermarket in the United States. It is made from grapes and has a slightly sweet taste that distinguishes it from other types of vinegar. Balsamic vinegar can be used to make salad dressings or marinades. Some people even drizzle it over ice cream.

You can create balsamic reduction by heating a small amount in a pot or saucepan over medium heat. Drizzle the glaze over meat, poultry, tofu, or seafood that has already been grilled or add it on during the very last minutes of cooking. If you don't have time to make the glaze, simply drizzle a small amount of the vinegar on your protein and enjoy.

TIP

Some people add a bit of brown sugar or honey to their glaze for sweetness, but you don't need to.

Spice It Up with Salsa

Salsa is a great condiment to keep in your refrigerator at all times. It has so many uses! Obviously, you can enjoy salsa on tacos and other Tex-Mex fare. But it also makes a great topping for protein!

Top your cooked chicken or skirt steak with a dollop of salsa. Or spoon it on top of tofu for a zesty, spicy flavor.

You can buy fresh salsa in the refrigerated aisle of the grocery store or if you want it to last a little longer, buy a jarred salsa in the middle aisles where you find other world foods.

TIP

You can also make your own salsa! Combine diced tomatoes, onions, cilantro, lime juice, and a bit of jalapeño for a spicy kick.

Use Yogurt to Make Meats Tasty

Greek yogurt can enhance the texture of your drier meats and proteins.

Prepare a yogurt sauce by adding fresh herbs, lemon juice, and garlic to plain Greek yogurt. Then let it sit for a few hours before serving it as a topping for grilled chicken or seafood.

You can also just use plain Greek yogurt as a marinade to add moisture to meat or as a dipping sauce.

Chapter **20**

Ten Grocery Shopping Tips for Macro Trackers

G rocery shopping can play a pivotal role in your success on the macro diet. The food you bring into your house is ultimately the food you will eat. Making nutritious choices in the store can help you to make choices at home that align with your goals.

But how we shop for groceries has changed significantly in recent years. Many people started to use online shopping during the COVID-19 lockdown and have continued to enjoy the convenience of e-shopping even after supermarkets opened back up.

Decide Between Online Versus In-Store Shopping

For sticking with the macro diet, there is no clear winner when it comes to online versus in-person shopping. But certain people will definitely benefit from each. You may want to consider the benefits of each style of shopping to see which group you think you fall into.

First, consider the advantages of going to your local market. The primary benefit of in-person shopping is that you can choose your own food. You can pick up that melon to make sure that it is ripe. You can chat with the baker to see when that loaf of bread was baked, and you can ask the butcher about the best way to prepare a certain cut of beef.

TIP

When you shop in the store, you have food experts at your fingertips who can help you expand your culinary repertoire and try new foods. Ultimately, if you find your macro meals to be interesting and delicious, you're likely to stick to your plan longer.

Other benefits of shopping in the store include

>> Comparison shopping is easier when you can see similar products side by side on the shelf.

>> It may be less expensive if the online venue charges for delivery.

>> Reading product information may be challenging on your smartphone and may be easier when you have the product in hand.

>> There are no order minimums, which can lead you to buy extra products just to avoid charges.

While shopping in the store can make choosing quality foods easier, it is less convenient than online shopping. Who doesn't love to be able to shop from the comfort of their couch? And if you have kids at home, there is no need to drag the little ones to the market or get childcare.

Other benefits of using your smartphone or laptop to buy groceries include

>> Budgeting is easier because you can see your bill before you place the final order.

>> Re-ordering is easy as many stores save your recent orders for you to review.

>> There is no waiting in line for check-out or other services.

>> You're probably less likely to make impulse purchases when you buy online.

>> You can add items to your cart over time. So, as you think of foods you need, you can put them in your virtual basket and then revisit it when you are ready to place your full order.

If you are a quick and efficient shopper and you tend to buy more fresh food, then going to the market might make more sense. But if you are short on time and you don't mind paying a little bit extra for convenience, then online shopping may be the best choice for you.

Regardless of how you choose to buy your food, these tips can help you to make healthy choices so that you can stock your kitchen with macro-friendly foods.

Make a List

Not only can a list help you to remember everything you need, but it may also help you to make more nutritious choices.

TECHNICAL
STUFF

According to a study published in the *Journal of Nutrition Education and Behavior*, using a grocery list is associated with healthier food choices and a lower BMI in people who are at high risk for obesity.

Making a list can also help you to navigate the store with ease and get your shopping done quickly and efficiently.

When you make a list be sure to include the quantity of each item that you need, so you don't buy more than you need or end up short on ingredients. Also, organize the list by department to make the shopping process more efficient.

Eat Before You Go

It isn't uncommon to go to the grocery store on the way home from work or from the gym. But if you're hungry when you roam the aisles, you are far more likely to make impulse purchases that are fueled by your grumbling tummy.

Have a quick protein- or fiber-rich snack before you go to the market so that you feel full and satisfied as you shop. This eliminates the possibility of making bad decisions based on hunger.

Shop the Perimeter

Most supermarkets (especially in the United States) are designed the same way: The perimeter of the store is where you will find fresh foods, such as produce, fresh bakery items, meat, seafood, and dairy. In many cases, these foods are more nutritious (and more delicious) than canned and frozen picks. If your budget allows for it, this is where you'll find the highest-quality goodies.

Head Down the Aisles

Yes, you should shop the perimeter of the market to get fresh fruits and vegetables and other less processed foods. But that doesn't mean you should skip the center aisles — especially if you are on a budget.

Some packaged foods are not only highly nutritious, but they are also much cheaper than their fresh counterparts. Consider canned or frozen fruits and vegetables, canned or dry beans, and other canned or packaged goods, like tuna. They are easier to store at home, and they last longer, making them more budget-friendly.

Choose Water Over Oil or Syrup

When you are looking at canned products, read the label to see what they are canned in. For example, some fruit is canned in heavy syrup that contains added sugar. Tuna that is packaged in water is much lower in calories and fat than tuna packaged in oil.

REMEMBER

When possible, choose foods that are canned in water rather than oil or heavy syrups to avoid consuming excess fat, sugar, or sodium.

Canned beans, for example, usually contain added sodium unless you specifically choose the ones labeled "low sodium" or "no sodium."

Eat the Rainbow

Many of us (myself included!) tend to buy the same fruits and veggies time and time again. A better way to approach the produce section is by challenging yourself to eat as many colors as possible. Nutrition experts often call this "eating the rainbow."

Look for colorful foods like bright red cherries, deep purple eggplant, orange peppers, green honeydew melon, yellow squash, and blueberries. By searching out different colors in the produce section, you learn to enjoy a greater variety of foods and gain all of the nutritional benefits that they offer.

Get Savvy about Grains

When you're shopping for starchy foods, opt for whole grains rather than refined or enriched grains when you can. You'll know that a food is made from whole grains by checking the ingredients list. Look for words like "whole wheat" or "whole grain" as one of the first ingredients. And be wary of other product claims on the package.

Keep in mind that if a product simply indicates that it is "made with whole grains," you don't necessarily know how much of the product is made from whole grains and how much is made from enriched or refined grains. In some cases, those products are made primarily from processed white flour.

TIP

Look for products that are made with 100 percent whole grain or 100 percent whole wheat when possible.

Whole grains contain more fiber, protein, vitamins and minerals than processed (enriched or refined) grains. Choosing whole grains rather than refined or enriched grains can help to lower your risk for certain diseases, including hypertension (high blood pressure), high cholesterol, and type 2 diabetes.

TIP

If you are using the macro diet to lose weight, the fiber in whole grains can help you stick to your plan. Fiber helps you to feel full longer after eating and may help to curb cravings.

Consider Big-Box Alternatives

Your local supermarket is likely to have the largest selection of products, but other options offer high-quality food as well.

For example, check out your local farmers market or food co-op. You might also want to look for a community-supported agriculture (CSA) organization.

When shopping from a CSA organization, you don't get to choose what fruits and veggies you get. So each box is a surprise, allowing you to taste and experiment with new flavors. This can be a huge win for macro trackers who prep meals. One of the major complaints about meal prepping is that the food can become boring if you prep the same meals all the time. But if you are provided with new foods to cook with each week, you'll be inspired to try new recipes and ideas. Plus, you support your local farmers, which is always a good thing.

You can become a member of a CSA by purchasing a share. Then local farmers provide produce and other fresh goods for you to pick up during the growing season.

Use Apps or Online Coupons

Dozens of list-making apps can help make grocery shopping easier. For instance, check out apps like AnyList, OurGroceries, or Mealime (which also has a meal planning feature) to make your grocery shopping process more streamlined and efficient.

TIP

If you have a smart speaker at home, you can also use it to keep a running grocery list for you. In some cases, the list can sync with your phone.

You can also add a coupon app to your smartphone. Apps like Rakuten, Savingstar, and others can help you to save a little cash when you buy nutritious foods.

Chapter **21**

Ten Macro-Balanced Snacks to Carry On-the-Go

Consuming a macro-balanced nutritious snack can help you to maintain energy levels and curb hunger between meals. For this reason, you'll see that each of the sample meal plans in Chapter 10 provides one or two snacks. Many online meal plans also include three meals and two snacks, one mid-morning and one mid-afternoon. But this shouldn't imply that snacking is necessarily the right choice for everyone.

TIP

You shouldn't assume that you *must* include snacks in your diet. Some people do better if they eat larger meals and skip snacking. In contrast, others do best consuming smaller meals and occasional snacks.

The science regarding snacking is inconsistent. Most research associates snacking with an increase in total daily caloric intake. But studies are mixed when it comes to how that affects body weight. Many studies show that even though snacking increases calorie intake, it is associated with a decreased risk of obesity and weight gain.

If you decide to include snacks in your plan, consider these portable options that require no refrigeration. Each provides a balance of protein, fat, and carbohydrates.

Hard-Boiled Eggs and Hummus

Hard-boiled eggs are one the most convenient snacks simply because they are easy to carry, easy to eat, and provide a healthy dose of protein (about 5 grams of protein — primarily contained in the egg white).

TIP

You don't need to keep hard-boiled eggs refrigerated as long as you eat them within two hours of removing them from the fridge (or you can carry them in a cooler bag).

The only issue with hard-boiled eggs is that they don't provide any substantial carbs. So, to make this a macro-balanced snack, you need to add some healthy carbohydrates. You can either grab a handful of berries to eat with your (whole) egg or scoop out the egg yolk and fill the yolk hole with hummus. This healthier version of deviled eggs is both savory and nutritious. To note, there is nothing wrong with egg yolks. Each yolk provides about 55 calories of (mostly unsaturated) fat. But if you swap it out for hummus, you get healthy fat along with carbohydrates (including fiber) for a more balanced snack.

Plant-Based or Meat Jerky

Beef jerky is another fan favorite when it comes to protein-rich savory snacks. A 30-gram piece of jerky provides about 10 grams of protein, a bit over 3 grams of carbs, and about 7.5 grams of fat. The primary downside is that it also provides more than 500 milligrams of sodium. Yikes!

You can look for lower fat and lower sodium alternatives if you're watching your salt intake. If you don't consume beef, turkey jerky is another option or a plant-based jerky alternative (although plant-based products contain far less protein).

Trail Mix

Trail mix is easy to pack, easy to carry, and super easy to nibble on when you're on the go. Most varieties provide carbs along with vitamins and minerals (usually from dried fruit) and healthy fats and protein from nuts and seeds. Some store-bought varieties, however, also may contain more added sugar than you are looking for.

You can assemble your own healthy trail mix at home by combining nuts and seeds that you enjoy (almonds, pistachios, macadamia nuts, sunflower seeds, or pumpkin seeds) combined with some whole-grain cereal or pretzels if you prefer. Then finally, add dried fruit for a hint of sweetness.

Protein Muffins or Brownies

Baked goods are a satisfying treat that can boost your energy levels and curb sugar cravings. Usually, however, they don't provide much protein. But you can change that if you bake your own muffins or brownies at home.

You can add protein powder to many muffin or brownie recipes to boost the protein content and make them a more macro-balanced treat. Some stores also sell protein-rich baked treats.

When you make protein-rich baked goods at home, replace one-fourth to one-third of the flour with a protein powder of your choice. Replacing more than that can result in a treat that is too dry and crumbly.

TIP

And if you like the convenience of muffins, but don't necessarily want a sweet baked good, consider making a savory muffin. Check out the "Savory Egg White Muffin" recipe in Chapter 15. Adjust it as needed according to your taste preferences.

Popcorn and Nut Mix

Popcorn is one of the healthiest and most satisfying salty snacks. It's also easy to pack and carry because it doesn't need refrigeration.

Popcorn is a whole grain, so when you enjoy this treat, you boost your fiber intake substantially. Your fat intake with popcorn will vary depending on how you prepare it.

TIP

Airpop the kernels to get less fat or cook it in vegetable oil to get more fat.

A single three-cup serving of popcorn does provide you with about 3 grams of protein, but if you want to boost that number, toss a handful of nuts into your popcorn bag.

Apple and Peanut Butter

An apple slice slathered with creamy peanut butter is the perfect sweet and salty snack. For many people, it tastes like a caramel apple. It also provides a nice macro balance to boost your energy and help curb hunger.

A small apple with two tablespoons of peanut butter provides about 275 calories, just under 8 grams of protein, and 32 grams of carbs (with more than 6 grams of fiber!). It also provides about 16 grams of mostly poly- and monounsaturated fat.

TIP

If you prefer to decrease your fat intake, opt for powdered peanut butter. It is easier to carry, and you can simply add water to make it creamy when you are ready to snack.

Tuna or Salmon and Crackers

Tuna pouches are readily available in almost every supermarket in the United States and Canada. They require no refrigeration and are fully sealed so they can easily be tossed into your purse or gym bag. Bring your own crackers or look on store shelves for tuna/cracker combo packs, which several large tuna producers make.

A Starkist tuna and cracker combo for instance, provides you with tuna, crackers, mayo, and relish to use if you prefer. You can chill it if you want, but refrigeration is not required as long as the packet remains sealed. Each kit provides 260 calories, 19 grams of protein, 25 grams of carbs, and 9 grams of fat.

Protein Balls

Protein balls are fun to make at home and a quick and simple snack to pack and enjoy. In most cases, no baking is required!

Visit Chapter 17 to find a recipe for pumpkin-flavored protein balls or find a recipe online for chocolate, peanut butter, or other flavors. Each ball is likely to provide about 4 grams of protein, about 8 grams of carbs, and about 4.5 grams of fat.

Roasted Edamame

You can make your own roasted edamame, or you can buy it pre-made. Either way it is a savory snack that requires no refrigeration and provides a balance of all three macronutrients.

A 1/3 cup serving of store-bought dry roasted edamame provides about 14 grams of protein, 9 grams of carbs, and 5 grams of fat.

TIP

If you don't like edamame, try roasting chickpeas. Visit Chapter 17 for a recipe.

Protein Bars

Protein bars are the original go-to protein snack. Over the years, they've landed in the nutrition doghouse because many of them are full of sugar and have more unhealthy fat than protein. But not all of them.

If you buy protein bars to carry as a snack, be sure to read product labels. Look for those that contain whole grains, unsaturated fats, and plenty of protein (you'd be surprised how little of them some provide). Try to avoid those that contain added sugar.

You can also make your own protein bars at home. In Chapter 17, you'll find a recipe for a nutty bar that is delicious and easy to make.

Chapter **22**

Ten Unexpected Benefits of Being on the Macro Diet

onsuming a balanced diet offers well-established health benefits. In Chapter 3, I go into detail about what you can expect when you change your eating plan to include a balanced ratio of protein, carbohydrates, and fat. I also include plenty of peer-reviewed studies to show you the extensive research that supports the link between diet and health. But eating a nutrient-rich diet full of foods you enjoy also supports you in other ways.

One of the most important things you can do to improve your health and longevity is to eat well. Food not only supports good clinical health, but it also supports a sense of well-being, connection with friends and family, and an overall sense of happiness.

Unlike other restrictive eating plans, the macro diet can help you enjoy food, community, and comfort. You can eat meals that make you happy but also take advantage of food combinations that help you reach fitness, health, or athletic goals. It's a well-rounded approach to nutrition.

In this chapter, I reveal some of the more unexpected advantages you might gain by going on the macro diet. As you notice these (or other) benefits throughout your journey, give yourself a pat on the back for making this investment in your health.

You'll Impress Your Friends in the Kitchen

You'll be most successful on the macro diet if you fine-tune your cooking skills. Maybe you already know how to boil an egg (which is important because eggs are a good source of protein and fat!), but if you take on meal-prep strategies, you'll not only learn to cook a wide range of other foods, but you'll be able to cook them in bulk.

TIP

If you're new to cooking, I've got you covered! Check out Chapter 8, which explains how to set up your kitchen like a pro. Then breeze through Part 5, which provides you with a wide range of breakfast, lunch, dinner, and even dessert recipes. Many of the recipes are simple enough for a kitchen newbie. Chapter 20 includes a list of helpful tips to make grocery shopping simple.

Eventually you'll be able to amaze your friends with skills like roasting buckets of vegetables, shredding pounds of chicken, or whipping up dozens of macro-friendly muffins. You may even get an offer or two to develop your own recipes or cook for others. As your skill level skyrockets, your kitchen prowess will blossom.

You May Out-Gym Your Gym Buddies

No doubt eating well brings your workouts to a new level. Nutrient-rich carbohydrates provide your body with energy, and protein provides your body with building blocks to build strong muscles. If you have a competitive group of workout buddies, your super-charged new self may inspire envy.

Have you been hiding in the back of your spin class? When you track your carbohydrate intake and increase your intake to provide more energy, you may feel inclined to hop in the front row. Have you been lagging at the back of your run group? Prepare to head to the front of the line! Has your elliptical game been lacking? It's time to try a new level. Eating nutrient-rich meals can give you the energy you need to up your game and even inspire others.

Your Muscles May Thank You

Maximizing protein in your diet can help you to gain mega muscle mass when combined with a targeted body-building program. But did you know that getting a balanced ratio of nutrients can also help those muscles feel better when your workout is complete? Fat, in particular, can help to improve recovery.

TIP

Research has shown that getting omega-3 fatty acids in foods like fish, nuts, or seeds can make your body feel better after you crush your workouts.

So, if you plan a macro-balanced post-workout snack that includes salmon, sardines, walnuts, or other omega-3 foods, your muscles are likely to recover with less soreness. The result? A happy, thankful body.

You Can Say Goodbye to Hanger Outbreaks

How many times has your mood tanked because your energy stores diminished? Have you snapped at your sweetie or snarled at a coworker because your blood sugar was low and you needed a snack? We've all been there. You get hungry and angry, and the *hanger* outbreaks follow.

On the macro diet, you plan balanced meals that help to keep your blood sugar levels steady throughout the day. You can also include macro-balanced snacks between meals to keep the hunger pangs at bay. In Chapter 17, you'll find recipes for snacks and sweets that can help you to stay satisfied all day long.

If you prep meals and snacks in advance, you'll always have nutrient-rich food ready to go. So, you can say goodbye to late-day mood swings and say hello to a calmer, steadier disposition.

You'll Become a Nutrition Whiz

The macro diet can be a bit time-consuming when you first start out because you need to learn nutrition basics. You'll familiarize yourself with the benefits of basic nutrients along with the foods that provide those compounds. But within a few weeks, you'll be surprised at how much you know about food and nutrition.

There will be no need to flip over every package or product at the grocery store. You'll remember how much protein is in a chicken breast (27 grams) or how much fat is contained in peanut butter (16 grams per two tablespoons). You'll become a walking (or jogging or cycling or swimming) encyclopedia of nutritional data for better health.

Your Diet Will Play Well with Others

One of the best things about the macro diet is that it is flexible enough to adapt to any lifestyle or food plan. That means if you change your eating style, you don't have to go off the macro diet. You can use your macro-diet savvy to support your new program.

TIP

The macro diet works alongside a vegetarian or vegan diet, a gluten-free diet, or other types of diets such as the Mediterranean diet, paleo diet, or DASH diet. In fact, you can use it to ensure you're getting a balance of good nutrition as you transition to a new food plan.

You'll Become the Envy of the Lunchroom

When you first start to prep meals, the focus should be on balancing nutrients. But if you're like most people on the macro diet, you'll eventually become a food prep master and accumulate all the bells and whistles that go with it, like lunch kits, specialty food containers, swanky smoothie shakers, and on and on.

So, when you bust out your lunch in your office breakroom, you may want to prepare yourself for the reaction you'll get from the brown-paper baggers beside you. Meal-prepped lunches in specialized containers *look* delicious. They often appear like something you pay big bucks for at the local health store. But you get the satisfaction of knowing that you made it at home (often on a budget!).

Want to make your coworkers envious in the lunchroom? Chapter 16 is full of yummy meal inspiration and recipes. In Chapter 8, I explain all about the different food containers and shakers you can use to keep your meals fresh.

You May Save Some Dough

You can expect to save money on the macro diet if you buy in bulk and prep your own meals. So, you might want to set aside a little extra space in your wallet for the extra bucks you'll be carrying.

When you plan meals in advance, you can take advantage of fresh seasonal produce and store sales to maximize your budget and still enjoy delicious meals. And you might eat out less often! Who wants to hit the fast-food drive-thru lane when you've got a hearty prepped meal ready to go? Eating your macro-balanced meal doesn't only save money, but it might also save you from consuming excessive empty calories.

So how will you spend your extra pennies? Meal prep containers are a great idea! Or perhaps you'll want to invest in a trainer to up your game at the gym. Sticking to a budget can help you to feel more empowered alongside an elevated sense of health and wellness.

You'll Banish Food Guilt for Good

The only thing that is off limits on the macro diet is feeling shame or guilt for eating. When you track your macros, you don't get a gold star for eating foods perceived to be healthy, and there is no punishment for eating foods that are perceived to be unhealthy.

On the macro diet, you may feel inspired to eat nutrient-rich foods that make you feel good. But you're also going to want to occasionally eat foods that offer less in terms of nutrition and more in terms of enjoyment or comfort.

Including both types of food in your meal plan is part of what makes the macro diet balanced and sustainable.

You Set Yourself Up for a Lifetime of Empowerment

The time you invest in the early stages of the macro diet will serve you well for a lifetime of eating enjoyment and nutritional wellness. You don't have to meticulously track your macros forever to take advantage of all it has to offer. You can! But it is not required.

When (or if) you decide that you want to stop tracking macros, the knowledge that you gain from learning about nutrition and your body's response to macros does not go away. You can refer to it throughout various changes in your life to use as you need. You might want to track your nutrition for a week here and there to see how your diet stacks up. You may want to take a month or two to increase a nutrient to reach a training goal.

The macro diet empowers you to make decisions that serve your goals and needs for a lifetime of good health and happy eating.

Appendix

Metric Conversion Guide

Note: The recipes in this book weren't developed or tested using metric measurements. There may be some variation in quality when converting to metric units.

Common Abbreviations

Abbreviation(s)	What It Stands For
cm	Centimeter
C., c.	Cup
G, g	Gram
kg	Kilogram
L, l	Liter
lb.	Pound
mL, ml	Milliliter
oz.	Ounce
pt.	Pint
t., tsp.	Teaspoon
T., Tb., Tbsp.	Tablespoon

Volume

U.S. Units	Canadian Metric	Australian Metric
¼ teaspoon	1 milliliter	1 milliliter
½ teaspoon	2 milliliters	2 milliliters
1 teaspoon	5 milliliters	5 milliliters
1 tablespoon	15 milliliters	20 milliliters
¼ cup	50 milliliters	60 milliliters
⅓ cup	75 milliliters	80 milliliters
½ cup	125 milliliters	125 milliliters
⅔ cup	150 milliliters	170 milliliters
¾ cup	175 milliliters	190 milliliters
1 cup	250 milliliters	250 milliliters
1 quart	1 liter	1 liter
1½ quarts	1.5 liters	1.5 liters
2 quarts	2 liters	2 liters
2½ quarts	2.5 liters	2.5 liters
3 quarts	3 liters	3 liters
4 quarts (1 gallon)	4 liters	4 liters

Weight

U.S. Units	Canadian Metric	Australian Metric
1 ounce	30 grams	30 grams
2 ounces	55 grams	60 grams
3 ounces	85 grams	90 grams
4 ounces (¼ pound)	115 grams	125 grams
8 ounces (½ pound)	225 grams	225 grams
16 ounces (1 pound)	455 grams	500 grams (½ kilogram)

Length

Inches	Centimeters
0.5	1.5
1	2.5
2	5.0
3	7.5
4	10.0
5	12.5
6	15.0
7	17.5
8	20.5
9	23.0
10	25.5
11	28.0
12	30.5

Temperature (Degrees)

Fahrenheit	Celsius
32	0
212	100
250	120
275	140
300	150
325	160
350	180
375	190
400	200
425	220
450	230
475	240
500	260

Index

adjusting for weight loss, 80–81

adjusting for weight maintenance, 82–83

total tech method, for creating meal plans, 159–160

trace minerals, 36

tracking app method, for creating meal plans, 159

traffic-light labeling system (UK), 98

trail mix, 291

trans fats, 32

traveling, 187–188

treats. *See* desserts, snacks, and treats

tryptophan, 23

tuna

with crackers, 292

Healthy Tuna Poke Bowl, 241

Tupperware, 258

turkey

Ground Turkey Sweet Potato Skillet, 232

Italian Meatball Casserole, 246

Savory Breakfast Burrito, 226

Spaghetti and Turkey Meatballs, 259

turkey sausage, in Savory Breakfast Burrito, 226

12/12 plan, 13

Twice Baked Potato Burgers recipe, 270

2,000-calorie, plant-based meal plan, 164–165

2,000-calorie 50/25/25 meal plan, 164

U

umami, 279

Underwood, Carrie, 20

unsaturated fats, 32, 33

urine color, 37

U.S. Center for Disease Control and Prevention (CDC), 41, 189

U.S. Department of Agriculture (USDA), 10, 20, 24, 83, 84, 87, 91, 93, 94, 95, 96, 103, 106, 133, 134, 151, 155

U.S. Department of Health and Human Services (HHS), 10, 24, 83

U.S. National Academies of Sciences, Engineering, and Medicine, 151

USDA FoodData Central (website), 102

V

valine, 23

vegan diet, 11

Vegan Southwest Tofu Scramble recipe, 222

vegetarian diet, 11

vitamin A, 36

vitamin B-6, 36

vitamin B-12, 36

vitamin C, 36

vitamin D, 34, 36

vitamin E, 36

vitamin K, 36

vitamins

about, 34–36

on nutrition label, 100

volume conversions, 302

W

walking, after eating, 185

Warning icon, 3

water

about, 36–38

adjusting to increase energy, 151

water chestnuts, in Thai Chicken Lettuce Wraps, 238

websites

Body Weight Planner, 79

Cheat Sheet, 4

for macro tracking, 102–103

National Alliance for Eating Disorders (NEDA), 60

Precision Nutrition, 103

USDA FoodData Central, 102

weight

adjusting TDEE for maintenance of, 82–83

checking, 142–143

conversions for, 302

reaching and maintaining a healthy, 46–49

weight gain

adjusting TDEE for, 81–82

alcohol and, 195

calories and, 15